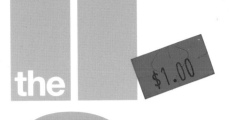

the 2 day diet

Diet two days a week.
Eat normally for five.

> 'Easier,
> longer lasting
> weight loss'
> *Red*

'Revolutionary and clinically prove
Good Housekeeping

Dr Michelle Harvie & Prof Tony Howell

About the authors

Dr Michelle Harvie and Professor Tony Howell work at the Genesis Breast Cancer Prevention Centre, part of The University Hospital of South Manchester NHS Foundation Trust. Genesis Breast Cancer Prevention is the only breast cancer charity in the UK entirely dedicated to prevention. Because weight is a significant factor in the risk of developing breast cancer, Dr Harvie and Prof Howell have spent years researching and developing the optimum diet to help people lose weight quickly and easily as well as keep off weight lost in the longer term. This incredibly effective diet is the result of their clinical research.

Dr Michelle Harvie is an award-winning research dietitian. For the last 17 years she has specialised in optimum diet and exercise strategies for weight loss and preventing breast cancer and its recurrence. Her findings have been published in many major scientific journals. She was awarded the British Dietetic Association Rose Simmond's Award for best published dietetic research in 2005, Manchester City Council's 2007 International Women's Day Award for Women in Science, and the National Association for the Study of Obesity Best Practice Award for best published obesity research in 2010.

Prof Tony Howell is Professor of Medical Oncology at the University of Manchester. He has specialised in treating breast cancer for over 30 years and now focuses on pharma- cological and lifestyle measures to prevent breast cancer. He is Research Director of Genesis Breast Cancer Prevention and has published over 600 scientific papers and book chapters, mainly concerning the biology of the breast and the treatment and prevention of breast cancer.

All author proceeds from the sale of this book will go to Genesis Breast Cancer Prevention (Registered charity number 1109839) www.genesisuk.org.

*This book is dedicated to four special
people who constantly inspire and
support me: my parents, Mary
and Terry Harvie; my wonderful
partner, Mark Garrod; and my
colleague and friend, Tony Howell.*
— Dr Michelle Harvie

*This book is dedicated
to my wife, Shelagh, for
her patience and support.*
— Prof Tony Howell

the

2

day diet

Diet two days a week.
Eat normally for five.

Dr Michelle Harvie & Prof Tony Howell

Vermilion
LONDON

7 9 10 8

This edition published in 2013
First published in 2013 by Vermilion, an imprint of Ebury Publishing
A Random House Group company

The Random House Group Limited Reg. No. 954009

Addresses for companies within the Random House Group can be found at
www.randomhouse.co.uk

The Random House Group Limited supports the Forest Stewardship
Council® (FSC®), the leading international forest-certification organisation.
Our books carrying the FSC label are printed on FSC®-certified paper. FSC
is the only forest-certification scheme supported by the leading environmental
organisations, including Greenpeace. Our paper procurement policy can be
found at www.randomhouse.co.uk/environment.

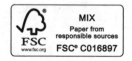

Designed and set by seagulls.net
and Colin Hall, www.typefunction.co.uk

Printed and bound by CPI Group (UK) Ltd, Croydon, CR0 4YY

ISBN 9780091948054

To buy books by your favourite authors and register for offers visit
www.randomhouse.co.uk

**All author proceeds from the sale of this book will go to
Genesis Breast Cancer Prevention (Registered charity number 1109839).**

The information in this book has been compiled by way of general guidance in
relation to the specific subjects addressed, but is not a substitute and not to be relied
on for medical, healthcare, pharmaceutical or other professional advice on specific
circumstances and in specific locations. Please consult your GP before changing,
stopping or starting any medical treatment. The authors and publishers disclaim, as far
as the law allows, any liability arising directly or indirectly from the use, or misuse, of
the information contained in this book.

contents

introduction

It won't come as a surprise to anyone reading this that we are getting fatter. Rates of obesity have reached epidemic proportions and worldwide there are now more overweight people than those who are a healthy weight. Despite massive government investment in healthy eating campaigns and any number of different diets promising effective weight loss, the number of us who are overweight just keeps rising.

But let's be clear, losing weight, even avoiding gaining it, is hard work in today's world. We are genetically programmed for an environment where food supplies are scarce and irregular, and we have to expend huge amounts of energy hunting it down – not for a world where food is available 24/7, we drive everywhere and are constantly tempted by supersized portions. With all this working against us it's hardly surprising that obesity rates keep rising. Losing weight is a struggle for anyone, however determined they are.

Our day-to-day contact with people desperate to lose weight means that we understand just how hard dieting can be, and the frustration and heartache that comes when you lose weight – then pile it back on. We also know how dangerous extra weight can be for your health. Our research is mainly focused on how excess weight increases the risk of cancer, but extra weight also contributes to heart disease, diabetes and dementia. As scientists with a commitment not just to our patients but also to improving the nation's health, we decided it was time to develop a research-based diet that would offer a different way to lose weight and keep it off.

With so many different diets on offer can The 2-Day Diet really make a difference? We believe that it can. The 2-Day Diet is designed to help you make the right choices, lose weight, change your habits and actively improve your health without leaving you feeling deprived. Our work with serial dieters has shown that this unique approach offers a real alternative for anyone who struggles to stick to a conventional diet. We were so impressed by the positive results of The 2-Day Diet that we wanted to make it available to everyone who is struggling – or who has struggled – to lose weight. The 2-Day Diet has paved the way to a slimmer, healthier future for many of our dieters. We hope it will do the same for you.

why The 2-Day Diet works

If you are someone who has tried, and failed, to lose weight, or you've shed the extra pounds, only to pile them back on again – this is the book for you. The 2-Day Diet is a brand new, research-based approach to weight loss, which can work for you, whether you've been struggling with your weight for years or have only just made the decision to lose weight. The 2-Day Diet is simple: you diet for just two consecutive days a week and eat normally for the other five days.

'I have never dieted and successfully kept the weight off – before I tried the 2-Day Diet. In fact I have always regained the weight and then usually extra, too. The 2-Day Diet is different – it's a lifestyle change that I can actually live with.' Marie, 33

We have become used to diet experts telling us that if we want to lose weight there are strict rules that we must follow every day. The 2-Day Diet approach turns all of that theory on its head. It's flexible, it's easy to follow and it will make you rethink your approach to dieting and find a different way to shift your unwanted pounds.

The idea of escaping the day-in, day-out restriction of a seven-day diet regime – dieting for just two days a week and eating normally for the other five days and still losing weight – probably sounds too good to be true. But it's not: our weight-loss research over the last 17 years with dieters, many of them serial dieters, shows that this new approach really can work, even when everything else has failed. The 2-Day Diet has been designed by research dietitian Dr Michelle Harvie, and, as well as delivering healthy, sustainable weight loss, The 2-Day Diet is nutritionally balanced to meet all your body's needs.

'Dieting on the two days was much easier than I had expected. I also found that I was much more mindful of my eating over the five normal eating days – I didn't want to undo all that good work!' Lizzie, 24

Warning

You should not attempt The 2-Day Diet if you are a child, a teenager, pregnant, breastfeeding, suffering from depression or have an eating disorder. The moderately high levels of protein in this diet may pose problems for anyone with kidney disease or anyone at risk of kidney disease. If you have diabetes, any other medical condition or if you are taking medication, seek advice from your GP before embarking on any diet and exercise programme.

If you are overweight, your main motivation for dieting may be to improve your self-esteem by regaining your true shape. You will lose weight on The 2-Day Diet, but you will also improve your health, protect yourself against disease and boost your energy levels. Research shows that losing even a small amount of excess weight (5 to 10 per cent of your body weight) can help reduce your risk of diseases such as type 2 diabetes, heart disease and some cancers. What's more, there's evidence to show that losing weight with The 2-Day Diet has the potential to have even greater health benefits than those gained by using a daily dieting weight-loss plan, as we will explain later.

The diet trap

In theory, losing weight should be easy. Eat less, move around more and the pounds should simply melt away. In practice, losing weight can be anything but easy. You might be able to lose a few pounds in the short term, but they soon creep back on again. Despite major public health campaigns and millions of pounds spent each year on diet products, the number of people who are overweight keeps on rising in almost all parts of the world, but particularly in the UK and USA. A 2007 MORI survey found that the average UK woman spends 31 years of her life on a diet, yet British women are now the heaviest in Europe. British men don't fare much better – 66 per cent are now overweight, positioning them as the second-heaviest in Europe. In 2010, 64 per cent of American women and 74 per cent of men were overweight. These figures occur alongside reports estimating that 108 million people in the USA follow weight-loss diets each year, spending $20 billion per annum on diet books, diet drugs and weight-loss surgery. It's clearly time for a new approach.

*'I can see and feel the weight loss, so I feel better
about myself. I don't feel so tired, I have so much
more energy in the evenings.'* Jane, 32

The story behind The 2-Day Diet

Our search for a different way to lose weight was driven by our work over nearly two decades with women diagnosed with, or at high risk from, breast cancer. We knew from our research and work done elsewhere that while being overweight significantly increases women's risk of developing breast cancer, losing weight – even as little as 10 lb (4.5 kg) – can cut that risk by between 25 and 40 per cent, compared with women who continue to gain weight, which is the norm[1]. The problem is that losing weight – and keeping it off – is extraordinarily difficult. Typically the dieters we worked with had already made between three and five serious attempts to lose weight. However motivated they were and however hard they tried, less than half of them managed to shed the weight needed to reduce their risk. Many enjoyed amazing short-term success and displayed extraordinary will power and determination, but, sadly, for most, the weight loss didn't last.

CASE STUDY: Anne

Anne's story is typical. Anne was desperate to lose weight, knowing that it was increasing her risk of developing the breast cancer that had already affected her mother, aunt and cousin, and her chance of developing type 2 diabetes, which had affected her father's side of the family. She had previously managed to lose 3 stone (19 kg) at a slimming group over a period of five months. This must have involved her eating 900 calories less than she normally ate each day for five months – 133,000 fewer calories in all! However, unfortunately, after all this effort, she regained most of the weight within four months.

Typically people stick with a diet for three to six months and lose around 1 stone (6.4 kg) in weight. The majority of people – 80 per cent – then put most of the weight back on again, while the remaining 20 per cent regain some weight but remain 8–12 lb (3.6–5.4 kg) lighter than their pre-diet weight[2].

So dieting isn't entirely in vain, since it can prevent you from gaining even more weight in the longer term. However, the process of constantly losing and regaining weight is demoralising, can lower your self-esteem and undermine subsequent attempts to lose weight. As many dieters are only too aware, dieting is a constant drudge.

'Thanks to The 2-Day Diet I feel less sluggish, less bloated, less tired after exercise, much healthier and my clothes now fit more comfortably.' Honor, 45

The size of the problem

- In 1993 53 per cent of adults in England were overweight (typically more than 1½ stone/9.5 kg above ideal weight) and 16 per cent were classified as obese (typically more than 3 stone/19 kg above ideal weight). The latest figures show that 59 per cent of women are overweight and 29 per cent are obese, while 66 per cent of men are overweight, with 25 per cent obese[3]. Very roughly, you can think of it in thirds: one-third of us are a healthy weight, one-third are overweight, while one-third are obese.

- UK women are the most overweight in Europe and UK men the second-most overweight[4].
- The NHS currently spends a massive £4 billion each year on weight-related health problems, which is forecast to rise to £6.3 billion by 2015.
- A 2011 Gallup survey reported that overweight workers in the UK are twice as likely to take time off work with poor health than healthy-weight workers.
- In 2006 the United Nations announced that for the first time the number of overweight people in the world exceeded those who were undernourished, with more than 1.3 billion people overweight and 800 million underweight.

Why diet for just two days a week?

Our initial studies between 1995 and 2005 used the conventional dieting approach and asked our Dieters to cut down calories on all seven days of the week. It became clear that many struggled with this standard approach, as they found themselves constantly having to think about their diet and what they were eating. By 2005, intriguing evidence of 'intermittent dieting', where calories are restricted for some days of the week, with a normal dietary intake for the other days, had started to emerge from scientists working in the fields of cancer and dementia. Papers published in 2002 and 2003 described how animals in the laboratory that were placed on intermittent diets developed significantly fewer cancers and less dementia than their counterparts that were following standard daily restricted diets[5,6]. Although these original stud- ies involved animals rather than people, the findings got us thinking. Most diets expect people to cut calories every day of the week, typically eating 25 per cent fewer calories each day and sticking to that regime. But what would happen if you did most of your dieting during two strictly observed days each week when you had around 70 per cent fewer calories on these two days rather than trying to cut down by the usual 25 per cent every day? Dieting for just two days each week could be a relief from the chore of having to diet every single day, which so many people struggle with. At the same time, two days is long enough to reduce your overall weekly calories, retrain your eating habits and, crucially, it seemed to have the potential to be more achievable. Would this approach be easier to follow than a daily diet? Could it be a better and more effective way to lose weight?

So back in 2006 we started researching two-day diets with funding from Genesis Breast Cancer Prevention and two other cancer charities (Breast Cancer Campaign and the World Cancer Research Fund), all of whom wanted to find more effective weight-loss approaches to help reduce cancer risk.

'The 2-Day Diet is a much more straightforward diet than any other I've been on. The two days "on" are easy to deal with if you put in a tiny amount of planning and doing it two days a week really makes you respect food on the days you aren't doing it. I lost 5 lb (2 kg) in the first 10 days and I don't have that "I'm on a diet" feeling.'
Matt, 41

Our first 2-Day Diet

The first 2-Day Diet we devised included two days of 650-calorie intake that only permitted milk, yoghurts, fruit, vegetables and unlimited low-calorie drinks such as water, tea, coffee and 'diet' drinks. The 650-calorie days were carefully designed to ensure that the Dieters met their nutritional requirements. Our 2-Day Dieters followed this diet for two consecutive days each week, eating a healthy Mediterranean diet (see page 70) for the other five days. They were then compared to a group of dieters who were asked to reduce their overall calorie intake by the same amount as the 2-Day Dieters, but by eating a standard, reduced-food intake every day of the week. A total of 107 women took part.

What we learned

We were encouraged by the results from this study. There was some evidence that, although the results were not substantially different from standard daily dieting, a two-day approach might be easier for some people to follow and have the potential for weight loss.

After six months 54 per cent of the 2-Day Dieters and 51 per cent of the daily dieters were successful and had lost at least 5 per cent of their weight. The 2-Day Dieters who stuck with the Diet for six months lost, on average, 1 stone 3 lb (7.7 kg) of weight, of which 13¼ lb (6 kg) was fat as well as 7.6 cm (3 in) from their waists, and 6 cm (2⅓ in) from their hips and bust. Some lost far more, with weight losses of 3 stone 4 lb (21 kg) and dropping at least three clothes sizes. For daily dieters, on average there was a 13 lb 9 oz (6.3 kg) weight loss, 10 lb 8 oz (4.9 kg) loss of fat and 5 cm (2 in) from the waist and bust.

Moreover, two-day dieting appeared to deliver greater health benefits than the daily diet. Both approaches were beneficial, but our 2-Day Dieters had a 25 per cent greater improvement in their insulin function than the daily dieters when we measured this five days after their restriction. They had a further 25 per cent reduction during and on the morning immediately after their two restricted days[7]. Insulin plays a vital role in regulating sugar levels in the body. Poor insulin function is a serious problem in modern life and is at the root of many weight-related diseases such as type 2 diabetes, heart disease, some cancers and possibly dementia. A large waist measurement is also associated with a greater risk of many of these diseases and our 2-Day Dieters also lost proportionately more weight from the waist than the seven-day dieters.

The intermittent diet approach could even be used for weight maintenance. Our 2-Day Dieters who lost weight switched to just one restricted day a week, kept the weight off and maintained the health benefits for the 15 months of the study – importantly, they maintained the reductions in insulin and cholesterol they had achieved with the diet.

Our new, improved 2-Day Diet

Using the lessons we had learned throughout our original diet research, we developed The 2-Day Diet, which forms the focus of this book.

Predictably the main downside of our original 2-Day Diet was that the food choices were so limited. Many of the Dieters on the trial found that only being able to have milk, yoghurt, fruit and vegetables was hard to stick to and only one-third of them were still following the diet by the end of a year. But we were so encouraged by the findings from our early research that we improved the Diet to include a greater variety of foods, and included more protein foods to make the Diet more satisfying, filling and easier to maintain long-term. Once again we tested The 2-Day Diet with two groups of women: one group doing the new, improved 2-Day Diet, the other a standard daily diet.

The feedback on the new, improved 2-Day Diet was even more impressive. Our most recent study, which followed women over three months' dieting and a month's maintenance found that six out of 10 women who set out to follow the Diet were successful, losing at least 10 lb (4.5 kg), compared to only four out of 10 following a standard daily diet[8]. Weight loss in this three-month study was slightly lower than our previous six-month dieters as this was a shorter spell of dieting. However, the weight loss we achieved was particularly encouraging as these Dieters were older, heavier and many had long-term weight and health problems.

The Dieters who managed to do at least 85 per cent of their two restricted days during the study (i.e. 20 out of their 24 days over three months) had the greatest rewards. On average they lost almost a stone (6.4 kg), over 10 lb (4.5 kg) of it fat, lost 5 cm (2 in) from the waist and hips and they dropped a clothes size. Again, some lost far more weight – they dropped two clothes sizes in three months, losing as much as 2 stone 4 lb (14.5 kg), 24 lb (10.8 kg) of it fat, just over 10.9 cm (4⅓ in) from the waist and hips and 8.9 cm (3½ in) from the bust. As before, our 2-Day Dieters had much greater reductions in insulin than seven-day dieters five days after their restricted days, and again they had the bonus of a further reduction of insulin during the two days when the calorie and carbohydrate intakes were actually reduced.

How The 2-Day Diet works

The 2-Day Diet provides clear guidelines about what you can eat on your two restricted 'diet' days. You eat foods that are high in protein, healthy monounsaturated fats (such as nuts), and fruit and vegetables, which are satisfying and reduce the feelings of hunger. Feeling fuller obviously makes you less likely to overeat. The 2-Day Diet is deliberately low in carbohydrates, which appear to make people feel hungrier[9]. On the other five, unrestricted, days you eat a normal, healthy, Mediterranean-style diet (see page 70).

The 2-Day Diet is designed to be:

▶ Low enough in calories to enable you to lose weight, but without leaving you feeling hungry.

▶ Nutritionally balanced so that all your vitamin, mineral and protein requirements are met.

▶ Easy to fit into a normal, busy lifestyle.

How is The 2-Day Diet different from other diets?
Cutting down for just two days is easier than cutting down every day.

Overall people found it easier to stick to two strict days than cutting calories every day. Although our seven-day and 2-Day Dieters both started well, with eight in 10 of them sticking to the diets during the first month, the seven-day diet became more of a struggle. After three months 70 per cent of 2-Day Dieters were still following their diet, compared to only 40 per cent of the seven-day group.

So why is a stricter regime easier to follow than a less-restricted diet? The answer seems to be precisely because it is strict. The 2-Day Diet has clear rules. From discussions with our 2-Day Dieters and previous research we know that as long as the diet is achievable, diets with restricted rules and limited choice can be easier to stick to than healthy-eating, low-calorie diets that have very flexible rules[10].

In fact, our bodies may even be biologically programmed for this 'intermittent' pattern of eating. The idea of having spells of normal intake and spells of restriction isn't new and some argue that it mimics the periods of food abundance and scarcity experienced by our hunter-gatherer Palaeolithic ancestors, who frequently went for long periods with very little food, interspersed with spells of eating more when food was available and abundant. This is a far cry from today's 24/7 food availability (and the fact that we don't have to hunt for it). Most people in the developed world have unlimited access to as much food as they want around the clock. In fact, many people don't even experience a proper overnight fast because they indulge in very late-night eating in front of the TV – perhaps a late snack at 2am, with breakfast only five hours later at 7am.

The 2-Day Diet retrains your eating habits

One reason why dieting is so hard is that it means breaking ingrained eating habits. Habits such as regularly consuming more food than we need, eating overly large servings, having too many fatty or sugary foods or habitual snacking (and often all of these). The 2-Day Diet helps you to change the way you eat. Losing weight is really very simple: it means cutting your overall calories by at least one-quarter and reducing your intake of high-sugar foods and saturated fat. For many people this is easier said than done. The 2-Day Diet gives you a much-needed break from your normal eating habits each week and helps you to develop vigilance and awareness of what you eat. These are vital skills, which put you on the road to being in control of what you eat and, therefore, your weight.

The 2-Day Diet develops your appreciation of food

Dramatically cutting calories for two days a week helps you to relearn how hunger feels and what a 'normal' serving looks like. You will learn to eat more slowly, appreciate smaller amounts and really enjoy your food on both your two restricted days and on the five unrestricted days. This will help you to rediscover how much food you really need, rather than the amount you have become used to eating. Our Dieters found that contrasting the two restricted days to their normal intake helped them identify what triggered them to eat – and to over-eat. If you're a serial dieter you may have become stuck in the low-fat, low-protein, high-carbohydrate pattern of eating, a combination promoted by many mainstream diets. While this approach may work for some, others find it difficult to maintain a daily low-calorie intake with these regimes, so they often find themselves overeating. The 2-Day Diet will help wean you away from these unhelpful patterns of eating.

The 2-Day Diet boosts your dieting confidence

For two days every week you have the opportunity to learn to resist temptation. This is a key dieting skill that you will need to practise until it becomes a habit. Being restrained on the two restricted days will give you the confidence to master your diet and food cravings and reinforce your desire to be in control of your diet on the other days of the week.

The success of The 2-Day Diet

The 2-Day Diet helps you lose fat rather than muscle

The best diets target fat and preserve muscle. Muscle doesn't just make you look and feel more toned, it's also the key to calorie-burning. Even when your muscles are resting they burn up to seven times as many calories as fat (see below). Dieters who followed the improved 2-Day Diet found that they lost proportionally more fat than the seven-day dieters, with 80 per cent of their weight lost as fat compared with 70 per cent for the daily diet group. If you follow what is called a 'very low calorie diet' (VLCD – around 500–600 kcal per day) you can lose only around 60 per cent of your weight as fat and 40 per cent as muscle. On The 2-Day Diet for every stone (6.4 kg) you lose you can expect to lose 11 lb (5kg) of fat and only 3 lb (1.4 kg) of muscle, compared with 8 lb (3.6 kg) of fat and 6 lb (2.7 kg) of muscle on some VLCDs. Another important point is that staying active while you're on the 2-Day Diet will help maximise your fat loss and limit your muscle loss even further (see page 118).

The 2-Day Diet may help to maintain your metabolic rate

Your metabolic rate, the rate at which your body burns calories, is affected by three things: your weight (the heavier you are the higher your metabolic rate because your body needs more calories to function); how active you are (active people burn more calories – see Appendix F, page 338); and the amount of muscle you have (the more muscle you have, the higher your metabolic rate because muscle burns seven times more calories than fat). One of the reasons why weight loss slows down when you diet is because your metabolic rate falls, typically by 10 to 15 per cent as you lose weight and have less muscle. Because the 2-Day Diet promotes fat loss and minimises the amount of muscle you lose it helps to limit the dip in your metabolism. The 2-Day Diet may also help burn a few more calories because of its high protein content – our bodies use 10 times more calories digesting and processing protein than for fat or carbohydrates. Although this doesn't have a major effect – it only burns an extra 65 to 70 calories a day – when you are trying to lose weight, small changes all add up.

You'll see rapid results

Losing weight can be hard work and dieters need to experience quick rewards so rapid weight loss is key to keeping you on track. There are no quick fixes – fat-burning is a complex process and it's hard to lose more than 4½ lb (2 kg) of fat a week – but you won't need to spend weeks on The 2-Day Diet before you see a difference. The 2-Day Diet performs better than seven-day dieting right from the start and sustains a greater rate of weight loss. Our dieters lost fat about one and a half times as quickly with The 2-Day Diet as with the conventional seven-day diet. After the first month our 2-Day Dieters lost, on average, 1–3 lb (0.5–1.4 kg) a week, which then slowed slightly. By contrast, the seven-day dieters only lost between ½ and 2 lb (0.3 and 1 kg) per week.

Our 2-Day Dieters lost more body fat mainly because, overall, they consumed fewer calories; however, they still shed more fat than expected, raising the possibility that they may have experienced a smaller drop in their metabolic rate as their weight decreased than the seven-day dieters – it is an interesting possibility, but one that is as yet unproven.

What happens to my body when I lose weight?

While you are dropping clothes sizes and/or tightening your belt a notch or two and feeling and looking healthier, major changes are taking place in your body. Your blood pressure and levels of harmful blood fats and hormones are all reducing, while favourable ones are increasing. These changes pave the way for a longer, healthier life. Eating too much will cause changes at the most fundamental level inside your body cells, leading to damage that increases your risk of cancer, type 2 diabetes and even early death. Eating less can halt and even reverse that damage.

How cells work

Your body is made up of millions of cells and although cells in different areas of your body have different specialist functions – in your brain, heart and bones for example – they all work in a similar way. At each cell's heart is a nucleus, the cell's control centre, which contains the genes you have inherited (your DNA). Genes are the blueprint for what makes you unique (your hair, eye and skin colour, for example). The activity of the cell is controlled both by the nucleus and by messages sent from within your body, which act on the cell via receptors on its surface. Cells produce their own energy supply and have their own power plants – called mitochondria. Each cell contains around 1,000 of these tiny bean-shaped structures that provide the energy the cell needs to do its essential work. Cells also produce waste products that need to be got rid of, so all cells also have their own waste-disposal units – known as lysosomes – which recycle all the damaged components of the cell.

What happens when you overeat and gain weight?

If you are overfed, then your cells will be too – and overfed cells don't work properly. When you take in more food than you need, levels of the hormones insulin and leptin rise in the body and send a barrage of messages to the cells, telling them to grow and produce lots of new cells. But when cells are putting all their efforts into growth and producing new cells, the lysosomes work less efficiently and the essential mainten- ance gets neglected, so waste builds up and damage fails to get repaired.

If this happened to your car it might carry on functioning for a while, but it wouldn't be long before it was off the road. When it happens in your body and you have increasing numbers of poor-quality cells that are not repairing damage and getting rid of waste, it becomes the starting point for many diseases, including cancer.

Overeating is also bad news for your cells' power plants – the mitochondria. They decline in number, become damaged and stop producing protective antioxidants. Like a worn-out battery, they start to leak harmful 'oxidising' substances, which can damage the cells and surrounding tissues. This damage causes inflammation, which if unchecked can lead to cancer, heart disease and diabetes.

As well as overfed cells becoming dysfunctional because of the barrage of signals they receive from hormones, overeating actually triggers certain genes in the cell to be switched on and others to be switched off. A recent study found that just five days of feeding healthy young men with a high-fat, high-calorie diet caused detrimental changes to their cells, by switching on genes associated with inflammation and cancer[11]. By contrast, other studies have shown that eating less and eating the right sort of foods, one example being resveratrol, the protective antioxidant found in fruits (especially grapes) and peanuts, can actually reverse these damaging changes and 'switch off' the harmful genes[12].

What is playing out in your cells when you overeat is similar to what happens to your body as you get older – so eating more than your body needs effectively speeds up the clock and ages you prematurely.

Why weight matters

- Being overweight increases the risk of heart disease, stroke, type 2 diabetes, dementia and more than 12 different cancers, including breast cancer, bowel cancer and cancers of the oesophagus (gullet), thyroid gland, kidney, womb, gall bladder, pancreas, malignant melanoma and cancers of the blood and immune systems, such as leukaemia, multiple myeloma, and non-Hodgkins lymphoma.

- People who are overweight are more likely to suffer from arthritis, indigestion, gallstones, stress, anxiety, depression, infertility and sleep problems.
- Being very overweight (3 stone/19 kg above your healthy weight) is as harmful to health as smoking and can reduce life expectancy by seven years. If you're very overweight and also smoke it can shorten your lifespan by 14 years[13].
- Being overweight limits healthy life expectation. In the UK women live, on average, to the age of 82, but their good health only lasts until their mid 60s, while men live to 78, with good health until the age of 64 often due to weight related illness[14].

What happens when you cut your calories?

Restricting your calories and losing weight helps to reverse the cycle of damage described above and gives your cells a spring-clean. Levels of insulin and leptin fall quickly (within 24 hours) when we eat less, so their signals that drive the cell to grow reduce and cells can put more effort into staying in top condition, repairing damage and removing waste. Damaged old mitochondria are removed and new ones are produced, which make more antioxidants, helping to reduce the inflammation in the cells and surrounding tissues. Lowering calorie intake also increases the number of waste-disposal units (lysosomes) and makes them more efficient at waste disposal. These rapid effects within 24 hours of dieting is one of the key reasons The

2-Day Diet has the potential to offer health benefits during the two restricted days each week.

Does this happen with every diet?

If you're overweight, cutting calories and losing weight is likely to produce all the beneficial effects described above. However, The 2-Day Diet, with the two restricted days, in combination with a five-day, Mediterranean diet, rich in plant chemicals, could be even more beneficial than a regular reduced-calorie diet. The two restricted days help to achieve a 40 per cent greater reduction in insulin than a standard calorie-reduced diet. This may be fundamental to the health benefits of The 2-Day Diet as excess insulin is one of the key drivers for the harmful impact being overweight has on cells and modern chronic diseases. There's also evidence that the lower the intake of calories, the better the waste disposal works so the low calorie intake on your two restricted days may have extra benefits. Restricting your calories may benefit your brain cells as well as those in the rest of your body. There's evidence from the work of Dr Mark Mattson, a neuroscientist at the National Institute on Aging in Baltimore, that dramatically reducing your calorie intake for some but not all days of the week could protect against Alzheimer's, Parkinson's disease and other degenerative brain conditions.

Exercise seems to have a similarly beneficial effect on reducing insulin levels, improving waste disposal and increasing the number of mitochondria. Exercise also has other beneficial effects – when muscles are being used they produce protective hormones and chemicals. These can help cut your risk of many diseases by improving your body's ability to deal with glucose, reducing inflammation and lowering levels of growth factors and hormones that are linked with cancer. They can also stimulate cells within the brain for optimal brain health.

What happens to worn-out cells?

Even healthy cells have a limited life and need to be replaced by new cells. This turnover is a natural process, but when your body doesn't work properly because of overeating and inactivity, this gets disrupted so that cells that have completed their useful life persist in the body – these worn-out cells, known as 'senescent' cells, are linked to cancer, heart disease and diabetes. Cutting calories has been shown to reduce the likelihood of these worn-out cells persisting in the body and ensure that they are eliminated.

CASE STUDY: Gillian

Gillian, 47, started The 2-Day Diet because she knew her weight was creeping up. Although only a stone (6.4 kg) over- weight, Gillian wanted to get down to a healthy weight and stay there. Gillian wanted a diet that didn't involve special foods or lots of planning, was simple enough to fit into her busy working life and still meant that she could go out for dinner with friends at the weekend. She did the Diet on her busiest work days and ate the bulk of her calories in the evening. 'Knowing that you're not depriving yourself all week makes this Diet so much easier and by the time you've finished your two days you don't feel like eating everything in sight, you just enjoy eating normally. I lost the weight quite easily and kept it off – I often do the Diet for one day a week to keep the weight off.'

Your questions answered

'Isn't The 2-Day Diet just "yo-yo" dieting?'

Yo-yo dieting and yo-yo weight gain and loss occurs when, despite trying to stick to a daily, restricted diet, you end up dipping in and out of it – sometimes dieting and sometimes lapsing.

People often worry that The 2-Day Diet is a type of yo-yo diet, where the Dieter loses weight for two days each week only to rebound on the days in between. The 2-Day Diet is different, because by carrying out the two-day restriction every week plus maintaining a healthy diet in between, your weight will steadily drop while following the plan.

'Why two days?'

We wanted to make a departure from the grind of dieting every day. The two days allow long enough to reduce your overall calorie intake, retrain your eating habits and it may have additional beneficial effects on metabolism and disease risk. It is also achievable.

'Do I have to diet for two consecutive days?'

We recommend that the two days are done together because many Dieters find the second day as easy, or easier than, the first as they have got into the habit of eating less. Doing the two days together also helps to ensure that you actually get round to doing the second day and it may have additional health benefits because it provides a prolonged period when the body is in a healthier metabolic state (see pages 15–19).

If you struggle to do the two days together each week, two separate days will be fine for weight loss, provided that you actually get around to doing them. In our research a small number of Dieters – just 5 per cent of the total – often did their two days separately and they still lost weight. You can choose which days of the week work best for you. Many of our Dieters opted for busy working days when they did not have much time to think about missing food, whereas others opted to do them at the weekend when they had more time to be organised. When you do the two days is up to you, but it's probably a good idea to try and keep to the same two days each week to establish a habit that you are more likely to stick to. However, the beauty of just having to diet for two days is that you can swap them, if necessary, to fit into your weekly schedule.

'I've heard that just eating once a day can work just as well?'

This may be the case if it means that you consume fewer calories overall. However, there are no obvious weight-loss or health benefits from going 24 hours without eating if you eat the same amount of food in one meal as you would have done in a number of meals throughout a day[15]. (See page 108)

'Don't people just binge on the five unrestricted days?'

If you like the idea of dieting for two days, but worry about overeating for the rest of the week you will be pleasantly surprised to hear that our 2-Day Dieters didn't binge on their unrestricted days. In fact most of them wanted to eat less than they normally did and this is part of the reason why The 2-Day Diet is successful. A key feature of The 2-Day Diet is that it appears to reset your appetite and retrain your eating behaviour for the whole week.

'Does it work for everyone?'

No diet works for everyone and this diet is no exception. The success of any diet is mainly due to whether people can follow it and keep it up over time. Our research showed that 60 per cent of the Dieters were successful, but 13 per cent of those who set out to do The 2-Day Diet had family, work or other personal issues which prevented them from sticking to it. Thirteen per cent of the women who tried it found that they couldn't adhere to it, while a further 14 per cent were trying to follow the Diet but only had partial success.

'Am I overweight because of my genes?'

People often wonder whether their struggle with weight is genetic and there's been much research over the past five years looking at how an individual's genetic make-up can affect their appetite and ability to store fat. However, although there clearly are genetic differences between people (32 weight-related genetic variants have been found so far), these are only thought to account for between a half and one per cent of the weight variations between different people[16]. So inheriting one of these genes probably means that you are a few pounds heavier than someone who does not. This is a new area of research. In the future we may be able to define the genetic make-up of dieters and identify those who may need extra support with weight loss or a different type of diet, but this is a long way off.

'Do my genes make it harder to lose weight?'

Although we haven't looked at this in relation to The 2-Day Diet, several recent studies have shown that genes make very little difference to people's ability to lose any weight, or the amount they lose. In a recent Spanish study, when dieters followed a 28-week diet and exercise plan, those with a particular type of gene lost 19 lb (8.6 kg), while those without the gene lost just 1.5 lb (680 g) more[17]. A recent Japanese study revealed similar findings. So the take-home message is that despite having the 'weight gene', dieters were still able to adhere to a diet and exercise regime and still lose weight[18].

'Do I have to follow The 2-Day Diet – can't I just cut calories for two days?'

We don't advise going without food or devising your own two-day low-calorie diet. The 2-Day Diet has been designed to keep you feeling as full as possible and to cover your nutritional requirements, with enough protein to limit loss of muscle mass, which is key to maintaining your metabolic rate and long-term weight-loss success. If you invent your own low-calorie diet you run the risk of it being both difficult to adhere to and nutritionally incomplete and it may not have the beneficial effect on muscle and metabolism.

'How will The 2-Day Diet fit in with family life?'

It should be easy to fit The 2-Day Diet in with family meals. On your two restricted days your family can eat the same as you, but they can add carbohydrates. For the five unrestricted days the healthy Mediterranean-style eating plan (see page 70) is suitable and beneficial for the health and well-being of the whole family.

'Are there benefits to following The 2-Day Diet if I am already a healthy weight?'

The first thing is to check that you really are a healthy weight, with a healthy level of body fat (see page 30). One in four people who have a healthy weight on the scales may be carrying too much fat around their waist. If you have a higher waist measurement than you should (see page 33) you will often also have two or more of the following:

▶ raised level of fat in the blood[a]

▶ raised blood sugar[b]

▶ raised blood pressure[c]

Even if the scales don't say that you're overweight, having weight around your waist puts you at higher risk of heart disease, type 2 diabetes and possibly certain cancers. If this sounds like you, then losing weight will be beneficial for your health.

If you have a healthy weight and waist measurement 2-Day Dieting is probably not a good idea as we don't know the impact of the Diet on individuals who are a healthy weight. However, having one restricted day a week may help you to maintain a healthy weight and prevent weight gain, especially if you are at a stage of your life when you might be particularly vulnerable to gaining weight. (See overleaf.)

'I am a vegetarian – can I still do The 2-Day Diet?'

The diet should work just as well for vegetarians as for those who eat meat and fish. The key is to make sure that you include enough protein and don't overload on carbohydrates. There are plenty of filling high-protein vegetarian foods and you will find plenty of vegetarian recipes for your two restricted days and for the five unrestricted days in chapters 9 and 10.

---

a. triglycerides: >1.7 mmol/L

b. > 5.6 mmol/L

c. >130/85 mm Hg

Risky times for weight gain

- Recent motherhood, when it is difficult to return to pre-pregnancy weight because of erratic meal patterns and lack of time to exercise. Please note that you should not do The 2-Day Diet if you are breastfeeding. Current guidelines state that once breastfeeding is established, overweight women can cut their calories by 500 kcal a day and do 30 minutes of aerobic exercise four days a week to lose around 1 lb (0.5 kg) a week[19].
- Settling down, co-habiting and getting married – when women may find themselves eating as much as their partners, despite normally needing far fewer calories.
- Giving up smoking.
- Times of stress and emotional upset.
- Studying or working long hours with many hours sitting at a desk or computer, erratic meal patterns, and often relying on high-calorie snack foods.
- Winter months – when we often crave higher-calorie comfort foods and are less inclined to exercise.
- Holidays and festive periods such as Christmas – when the average weight gain is 5 lb (2.2 kg)[20].
- Some drugs can cause weight gain, including steroids, oral contraceptives, betablockers and some anticonvulsants and antidepressants.

How much weight will I lose?

The average and maximum weight you can lose in the first three months on The 2-Day Diet is shown below. As you can see, the health benefits occur very rapidly within this first month of dieting.

The drops in cholesterol and blood pressure indicate a reduction in the risk of heart disease of 25–30 per cent, and the risk of stroke by 35–40 per cent. To maintain these benefits you need to maintain your lower weight and healthy lifestyle behaviours (see chapter 7).at

What can be achieved in the first three months of The 2-Day Diet							
	Month 1		Month 2		Month 3		Month 4	
	Average	Max	Average	Max	Average	Max	Average	Max
Weight	-6 lb (-2.7 kg)	-14½ lb (-6.6 kg)	-4 lb (-1.8 kg)	-12 lb (-5.4 kg)	-3 lb (-1.4 kg)	-8¾ lb (-4.0 kg)	-13 lb (-5.8 kg)	-32 lb (-14.5 kg)
Body fat	-4½ lb (-2 kg)	-11 lb (-5 kg)	-3½ lb (-1.5 kg)	-9½ lb (-4.3 kg)	-1¾ lb (-0.8 kg)	-10 lb (-4.5 kg)	-10 lb (-4.5 kg)	-24 lb (-11 kg)
Waist	-2.6 cm (-1 in)	-6 cm (-2⅓ in)	-2 cm (-¾ in)	-8.5 cm (-3⅓ in)	-1 cm (-⅓ in)	-8 cm (-3 in)	-6 cm (-2⅓ in)	-19 cm (-7½ in)
Insulin change	-10%	-74%	1 to 3 months Average -7% Max. -66%				-12%	-76%
Cholesterol change	-6%	-34%	1 to 3 months No change				-6%	-34%
Blood pressure change	-11%	-38%	1 to 3 months No Change				-11%	-40%

Summary

▶ The percentage of adults who are overweight in England is one of the highest in Europe and is increasing; 59 per cent of women and 66 per cent of men are overweight. In the USA 64 per cent of American women and 74 per cent of men are overweight. Despite large amounts of time and money invested in diets many people struggle to achieve and maintain successful weight loss.

▶ The risk of diseases such as cancer, heart disease, diabetes and dementia increase with increased weight.

The 2-Day Diet

▶ The 2-Day Diet is a new, nutritionally balanced approacho dieting designed to retrain your eating habits, maximise weight loss and preserve calorie-burning muscle.

▶ The 2-Day Diet involves restricting yourself to eating protein, healthy fats, fruit and vegetables for two consecutive days each week. For the remaining five unrestricted days you eat abalanced Mediterranean-style diet.

▶ The 2-Day Diet appears to achieve better and more rapid weight loss, greater health benefits and, for some Dieters, better long-term success than a standard, everyday restricted-calorie diet.

2

do I need to lose weight?

If your favourite jeans feel a bit too close-fitting for comfort, or you've found yourself moving up a clothes size or two, the answer to the question about whether you need to lose weight might be obvious. But how can you tell whether your weight gain could actually be harmful to your health? Health problems arise from carrying too much fat – especially if you have fat stored in the wrong places, such as excessive fat in the abdomen or muscles. So just looking in the mirror or standing on the scales may not immediately tell you the answer.

'I decided to do the diet because of the way I felt – sluggish, my joints were twingeing, especially my hips and knees. I want to be more energetic as I get older. I want to be healthy.' Jean, 61

What's your Body Mass Index (BMI)?

Start by working out your BMI – the most common way of measuring whether or not someone is overweight. You need to take height into account because someone who is 12 stone (76 kg) and 1.52 m (5 ft) tall is overweight, whereas for someone who is around 1.82 m (6 ft), 12 stone is an ideal weight.

BMI is calculated as your weight (in kg) divided by your height (in metres) squared. So, for example, the average women in the UK weighs 11 stone 3 lb (71.2 kg) and is 1.62 m (5 ft 4 in) tall, which means she has a BMI of 27.1 – above the healthy range of 18.5–24.9. A BMI of 25–29.9 is classified as overweight with increased health risks and a BMI of 30 or more is classified as 'obese', with even greater health risks. The healthiest BMI is actually around 20–22. A BMI higher than this can start to increase your risk of cancer and other diseases. The higher your BMI the greater your risk.

But BMI is only part of the story – two people can be the same height and weight, but carry vastly different amounts of body fat. A woman with a BMI of 27 who does no exercise could have as much as 43 per cent of her weight as fat, while another might be an athlete with lots of muscle and only 19 per cent of her weight as fat. So while they both have a BMI that puts them in the 'overweight' category, one has three times the amount of body fat and, as a result, very different health risks.

How to measure your body fat

If possible, try to measure your body fat as this will give you the best indication of how overweight you are. You can buy yourself a set of stand-on scales or a hand-held monitor that will measure your body fat for around £30–£50, but you'll also find these available to use in some pharmacies and shopping centres. These machines work by passing a tiny, imperceptible

do I need to lose weight?

Body Mass Index (BMI) Ready Reckoner

Height (m)

Weight (kg) — vertical axis on left, values ranging from 115 down to 26.

Height (m) column headers: 1.36 1.38 1.40 1.42 1.44 1.46 1.48 1.50 1.52 1.54 1.56 1.58 1.60 1.62 1.64 1.66 1.68 1.70 1.72 1.74 1.76 1.78 1.80 1.82 1.84 1.86 1.88 1.90 1.92 1.94

Weight (Stone, lb) — vertical axis on right.

Height (feet & inches)

Feet: 4 4 4 4 4 4 4 4 5 5 5 5 5 5 5 5 5 5 5 5 6 6 6 6

Inches: 5½ 6¼ 7 8 8¾ 9½ 10½ 11 11¾ ½ 1½ 2¼ 3 3¾ 4½ 5 6 7 7¾ 8½ 9 10 11 11¾ ½ 1¼ 2 2¾ 3½ 4½

Legend

- ▨ Obese
- ☐ Overweight
- ▨ Healthy Weight
- ▨ Underweight

31

electric current through your body. Your lean tissues (i.e. muscle and organs) contain mainly water and electrolytes that conduct this current, whereas fat, which contains little or no water, isn't a good conductor and impedes the current. By measuring how much lean tissue you have, the monitor estimates how much fat you have from your overall weight (i.e. total weight – lean-weight = fat weight). Stand-on scales, which send a current through your lower body, are more accurate than hand-held monitors that just measure your arms, although they are not foolproof. They will underestimate your fat levels if you have extra fluid in your body, for example for women around the time of their period, or if you have internal metalwork such as metal joint replacements. They will also overestimate your fat level if you are dehydrated.

For best results use a body fat monitor at the same time of day, once a week, ideally first thing in the morning. Wear minimal clothing, empty your bladder before use and avoid using the device straight after exercising, drinking alcohol or eating. Please note that you shouldn't use body-fat meters if you have a pacemaker.

Alternatively you can use our Body Fat Ready Reckoner (see Appendix A, page 314), which estimates your body fat from your weight, height, age and sex.

As a general guide, women should have between 20 per cent and 34 per cent of their body weight as fat and men should have between 8 per cent and 25 per cent[1].

'I had to do something – I was constantly worrying about my weight, I had no interest in clothes and I was always planning a diet. Something had to change.' Sandra, 49

Check your waistline

For certain health risks, for example, heart disease and diabetes, your waist measurement may be even more important than your weight. Some people gain weight on their bottoms and thighs (making them classic 'pear' shapes), while others pile it on around their waist (making them classic 'apple' shapes). Men are typically more apple-shaped than women, especially if they have 'beer bellies', but as women get older they tend to gain weight around their middles rather than their hips and thighs. Contrary to what many people think, this weight re-distribution can start to happen before the menopause[2].

If you're an 'apple', with extra fat around your middle, the odds are that you also have a lot of extra fat stored on the inside, around the vital organs inside your abdomen. This internal fat is very dangerous for your health, causing inflammation in the body, which in turn increases the risk of type 2 diabetes, heart disease, stroke and possibly some cancers. This intra abdominal fat' can be seen clearly in the scans below.

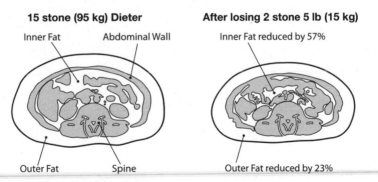

15 stone (95 kg) Dieter — After losing 2 stone 5 lb (15 kg)

Inner Fat — Abdominal Wall — Inner Fat reduced by 57%

Outer Fat — Spine — Outer Fat reduced by 23%

Here are two scans taken across the abdomen using magnetic resonance imaging. They are taken on the same person before and after losing 2 stone 5 lb (15 kg). You can see that the right-hand scan after dieting is smaller than the left. The white areas are fat. You can see the fat as a layer under the skin and also in the abdomen. The grey areas are muscle and bone in the spine and the organs and bowels in the abdomen. This 40-year-old woman, who had a strong family history of breast cancer, lost 2 stone 5 lb (15 kg) over the six months between the two scans. This represents about one-sixth (15.5 per cent) of her overall body weight and her BMI changed from 32 to 26.

In general you have a higher risk of health problems if your waist is too large. As a guide, your waist should be less than half of your height. Our research on 105,000 women found that women with a waist measurement of 90 cm (36 in) or more had a 40 per cent greater risk of breast cancer, compared to women with waist of 73 cm (29 in)[3]. Use the chart below to check your waist measurement. It will help you to work out if you have too much inner fat and need to lose weight.

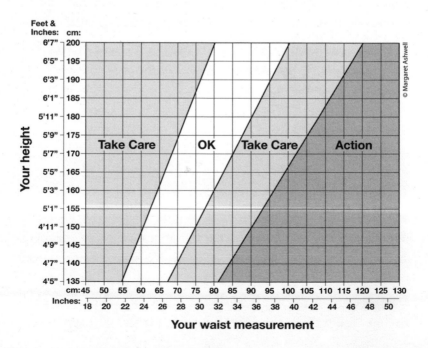

'My joints ached when I woke up.
I was breathless if I had to run up a flight of stairs. I
couldn't fit into any of my clothes, my arms were wobbly,
I looked frumpy, old and middle-aged... shall I go on?'
Charlotte, 41

Commit to change

We know from the experiences of our Dieters that commitment is the key to making The 2-Day Diet work for you, even if other diets have failed. Making changes to your diet and lifestyle isn't easy, but being committed, motivated and prepared for the challenge ahead is vital to your weight-loss success.

Why do you want to lose weight?

There may be lots of reasons – to improve your health, reduce your chances of developing cancer or to have more energy for playing with your children or grandchildren. For many of us the big motivator is to look better, feel more confident and be able to wear nicer clothes. We often find that many dieters worry that this is self-indulgent and not a valid reason for weight loss – and as a result they find it hard to admit that this is their motivator. Whatever your motivation, it's important that you are losing weight for yourself rather than to please or placate someone else.

List your reasons for wanting to lose weight and the positive benefits you stand to achieve for your health, well-being and self-esteem. Then write 'I am committed to losing weight because...' and add your reasons. Put this somewhere where you will see it every day – on your office wall, the fridge or on the kitchen notice board. It will give you a daily reminder of why you are doing the diet and will help you when you are having a difficult day or feel like giving up.

'I'm due to turn 50 this year and I've dieted on and off for most of my adult life. I was just fed up with it all. I needed something that will last.' Vicky, 49

Is now the right time to diet?

Losing weight isn't just about will power. It's hard to take on any new challenge if you're too stressed, have lots of other changes happening in your life or you haven't got the support of the people around you. Ask yourself:

▶ How are my stress levels – do I feel in control of my life?

▶ Do I have the support of my friends and family?

▶ Can I persuade any of my friends, colleagues and/or family to do The 2-Day Diet with me for moral support and motivation? A bit of gentle competition can spur you on when you are dieting, keep you on track and focused on your goal.

▶ Am I confident that I will be able to make the changes to my diet?

▶ Can I see a way to plan meals and fit regular exercise into my daily life?

If you answer 'yes' to most of these questions, you're probably ready to get going on The 2-Day Diet. If not, it's time to think about ways to manage your stress levels and find the support you will need to make The 2-Day Diet work for you.

Getting the support you need

If you've been on a diet before, you will know that there are plenty of diet saboteurs out there; the partner who wants you to stay 'cuddly'; the friend who persuades you to eat that piece of cake 'just this once'; or the mum who tells you that you were never designed to be thin. Having the wholehearted support of your nearest and dearest can really make a difference to your diet success, so it is important to bring people on board from day one. Watch out for sabotaging behaviour – tempting you with forbidden foods, critical comments about how the Diet has 'changed' you, suggestions that you're 'not one of us' any more. These are often difficult issues and may involve friends or family who are overweight themselves and don't like to see someone doing what they should be doing. Or they may be partners who feel threatened by seeing their other half gaining confidence and becoming more attractive to others. It is tempting to try to ignore such comments; however, we have found that when dieters clearly explain their reasons for trying to lose weight and actively ask for people's support, the sabotage stops and is replaced by support. One of our dieters described how taken aback she was by her work colleagues' negative response to her dieting. 'They used to put chocolates and biscuits on the table and I was amazed by their response to me not wanting a chocolate biscuit, so I actually stood up and said look, cards on the table, and explained that I was dieting to reduce my risk of breast cancer. When I explained things they were positive and supportive, but it took me doing that for them to really engage in it.'

How do you feel about yourself?

Very few of us are totally happy with our size, shape or how we look, especially when we are overweight. But for some people these negative feelings are so powerful that they have a major impact on their confidence, self-esteem and the way they live their lives. It's crucial to acknowledge and address negative feelings before you start dieting because if you feel bad about yourself it can be even harder to make healthy lifestyle changes and lose weight.

If this sounds like you, give yourself time to stop and think carefully about how you see yourself and how your body image affects your day-to-day life and your ability to cope with new people or situations. It might take some time to think through the issues, but it will be time well spent and can only improve your chances of success. Try to focus on what you like about yourself as a person, the things you like about your appearance and the positives about your life rather than dwelling on the things you want to change.

Manage your stress

Food and drink can become a refuge when life gets on top of you, so stress can be a major player in the struggle to control weight. The first step is to identify what causes stress in your life and learn to recognise its tell-tale symptoms. You then need to find ways to reduce and manage your stress levels without resorting to food. The following steps may take a bit of time to consider, but it is time well spent.

1. Make a list

List the main stresses in your life. They may include work issues, relationships, separation, family demands, bereavement, money problems, juggling too many roles, spreading yourself too thinly, the general pace of life, fear of failure, lack of support, feeling guilty about taking time and space for yourself or practical things such as driving a car. Issues surrounding diet, weight, exercise and health are often a source of concern and guilt.

2. Learn to recognise your stress symptoms

Common signs include feeling that you can't switch off, are not coping well, are not being efficient, feeling wound up, panicked, unable to support others, feeling you are letting people down. You may feel tired, develop headaches, feel tense and achy, have problems sleeping or become irritable and anxious. You may find yourself eating more, or sometimes less, or drinking more alcohol than you usually do.

3. Develop your coping strategy

How you manage stress will depend on what works best for you. Look at the list of stressful things in your life and take a long, hard look at how you can reduce the pressure on yourself. Put your stresses in order of priority, with the 'must do's' at the top. Starting at the bottom of the list, think about what you might be able to cross off or delegate to other people. If life feels out of control because of piles of unpaid bills or clutter everywhere, make a decision to tackle it, a little at a time. Getting organised can be a great antidote to stress. And if you're the kind of person who is always ready to step in when other people need help – and end up feeling overloaded as a result – start saying 'no'. It will be hard at first, but the more often you do it, the easier it gets.

Find ways to make time for yourself. If you feel that you're 'running on empty', try to carve out some space in the week (ideally every day) to do whatever helps you to wind down. What we do to de-stress is very individual and what works for you may not appeal to someone else. Some of the best ways to destress are also the simplest: get outside and walk – even a 10-minute walk, ideally in natural light, will help to recharge your batteries; join a choir – singing has been shown to help reduce stress and improve mood[4]; have a laugh – watch a funny film, read an amusing book, spend time with friends who make you laugh; book yourself a spa day, massage or facial; go to a football match; catch up with friends who make you feel good (not the ones who make endless demands and sap your energy); turn up the volume and listen to your favourite music at full blast; invest in a relaxation tape or find a yoga or meditation class; make time for sex in your life.

Plan for success

As well as listing the benefits of losing weight, spend some time thinking about the challenges you might encounter along the way. If you've dieted before, you probably already have a good idea of the kind of problems that you are up against, whether it's losing motivation, giving in to temptation or feeling unsupported by your nearest and dearest. By acknowledging and addressing these issues now, you will be ready to deal with the problems if and when they arise. Use a table like the one below to help you.

Benefits of doing The 2-Day Diet:	Problems I may encounter on The 2-Day Diet:
e.g. I will lose weight, feel better about myself, have more energy	e.g. Other people may try to persuade me to break the diet; being tempted to snack in the evenings
Benefits of not doing The 2-Day Diet:	**Problems with not doing The 2-Day Diet:**
e.g. Being able to eat whatever I want and whenever I want	e.g. I may gain more weight; I will feel more sluggish and have less energy

Set your weight-loss goals

Your goal is to reach your ideal weight as quickly as possible, but, as every dieter knows, weight loss takes time. We know that good, rapid weight loss from day one boosts motivation and is a real incentive to carry on[5] – and the good news is that you can expect to see results quickly with The 2-Day Diet (see page 15). We found that our 2-Day Dieters not only lost weight about 50 per cent more quickly than those on an everyday diet, but they were also able to change their eating patterns and reduce their appetite, which helped them to keep to the diet and maintain motivation.

It's good to have high ambitions, to aim to get back into a size 10 pair of jeans, or 32-inch waist jeans for men, or look good in a swimming costume/trunks. However, it pays to be realistic about how much weight you will lose and how long it will take to lose it. As you may recall, our 2-Day Dieters initially lost, on average, between 1–3 lb (0.5–1.4 kg) a week, which slowed down slightly so that by the end of three months they had lost, on average, 13 lb (5.8 kg) and some had lost far more. When it comes to weight loss, it's slow and steady that wins the race and our 2-Day Dieters who stuck with The 2-Day Diet were the biggest winners and saw the biggest changes. So there's absolutely no reason why your weight-loss goal shouldn't be ambitious, especially if you're convinced that you can rise to the challenge and keep going. However, your goal also needs to be realistic and achievable.

In the short term
– the first three months

Lose 5–10 per cent of your weight

It may not sound much, and it's almost certainly far less than your overall goal, but if you can initially lose and keep off just

5–10 per cent of your weight – that's 9–18 lb (4–8 kg) if you weigh 12 stone 8 lb (80 kg). You may well see instant health benefits and will be reducing your risk of type 2 diabetes by 60 per cent[6], as well as cutting your risk of heart disease by 70 per cent[7]. Our work has also shown that this amount of weight loss cuts the risk of breast cancer by 25–40 per cent[8].

Some people will lose the weight faster than others. If you follow The 2-Day Diet correctly, most of the weight you lose will be fat and, crucially, you should lose a substantial amount of the fat stored around your vital organs in the abdomen. This is important as this intra-abdominal fat potentially poses the biggest threat to your health. Research has shown that losing relatively small amounts of weight (10 per cent) can help you lose 40 per cent of the fat stored in your liver (which is partic- ularly dangerous for your health)[9]. Your liver is the HQ for your body's metabolism – it regulates the levels of circulating fat and sugars. Because a fatty liver doesn't work efficiently, you can have higher blood levels of sugar and fats, which in turn can lead to heart disease, diabetes and cancers as well as permanent liver damage.

Your longer-term goal

Everyone is different and it will be up to you to determine your personal weight-loss goal and how you set it. You might want to aim for your chosen ideal weight or want to get back to a weight that felt right for you in the past. Don't be scared to be ambitious, as long as your goal is realistic and achievable. Many of our 2-Day Dieters more than fulfilled their weight-loss ambitions. It may help to define small interim goals for two- or three-month blocks that you have a real chance of achieving. This will boost your confidence and your motiva- tion to arrive at your destination goal.

Summary

▶ Do your groundwork. Calculate your Body Mass Index, measure your waist and work out your body fat level before you start The 2-Day Diet – to help you know how much weight you need to lose.

▶ Be clear about your reasons for wanting to lose weight and make sure you have the right support to start on a diet to give yourself the best possible chance of success.

▶ Set yourself clear short-term and long-term weight-loss goals so that you know what you are aiming for.

▶ Don't forget! Even losing small amounts of weight can substantially improve your overall health and lower your risk of disease.

3

how to do the two restricted days

In this chapter we're going to explain how to do your two restricted days on The 2-Day Diet. We've designed this diet to: reduce your appetite, so that you are less likely to feel hungry; meet all your nutritional requirements, so that you won't need to take supplements; and ensure that you lose as much fat as possible and preserve as much calorie-burning muscle as you can. If you are vegetarian, The 2-Day Diet will also work for you, since vegetarian choices of protein foods are just as, and possibly more, filling than meat.

Warning!

Don't be tempted to devise your own two-day low-calorie diet. It will not only be harder to do because it will almost certainly leave you feeling hungry, but a 'made up' diet that isn't nutritionally balanced is unlikely to deliver the same health or weight-loss benefits as The 2-Day Diet.

The beauty of The 2-Day Diet is its simplicity and the fact it only has to be done on two days of the week, ideally consecutive: two restricted days are easy enough to fit into the busiest lifestyle. You don't have to count calories or go hungry. All you need to do is to stick to the recommended foods listed, making sure that you include the minimum recommended servings, but that you don't exceed the maximum. By using these simple rules to retrain your eating habits The 2-Day Diet will help to put you back in control of what you eat and help you lose weight.

The 2-Day Diet

▶ For two days each week you are allowed foods that are high in protein, healthy fats, low-fat dairy foods, some vegetables and fruit. There's no calorie-counting to do; just use the Ready Reckoners (see pages 328–331) to check the minimum and maximum number of servings of each type of food you can eat, which are stated for men and women.

▶ For two days your intake of carbohydrate is limited to around 50 g per day. This is because research shows that carbs make you hungry! With minimal carbs your body quickly shifts from storing fat to burning it. It is the by-products of this fat-burning, partly ketones and partly other by-products, that suppress your appetite.

▶ We recommend that you do your two restricted days back-to-back to get the full benefits of the Diet. Our research found that doing the two days together makes dieting easier and ensures that you actually get around to doing the second day. It may also have extra health benefits.

'The diet has totally transformed my eating habits and I actually look forward to my two restricted days!' Kate, 27

How much can I eat?

We haven't imposed a strict calorie restriction on the two restricted days because we found that The 2-Day Diet is so satisfying that Dieters naturally restrict the amount they eat. We have given you a guide to the maximum number of servings of each type of food, to help reassure you that you aren't eating too much. Remember that these are *maximum* allowances and you don't have to eat the maximum amount – most of our Dieters didn't. Dieters often worry that if they don't eat enough they won't lose weight, but this is definitely not the case. However, it is important that you have enough protein and electrolytes on the two restricted days. For this reason we recommend that you have at least the minimum recommended amounts of protein foods and that you try to have your dairy, fruit and vegetables, but beyond this only eat as much as you need and listen to your body. If you're not hungry, eat less! You will find details on all the serving sizes in Appendix B on pages 316–321 at the back of the book.

'I thought The 2-Day Diet was going to be hard but it was so much easier than I expected. The scope of foods is vast and you can vary your meals so you don't get bored with what you are eating.' Kerry, 32

On each of your two restricted days of The 2-Day Diet you can consume:

▶ Protein foods (i.e. chicken, fish, eggs, lean meat): a maximum of 12 servings for women and 14 for men.

▶ Fats (i.e. rapeseed, olive oil, nuts or avocado): a maximum of 5 servings for women and 6 servings for men.

▶ Dairy: 3 servings.

▶ Fruit: 1 serving.

▶ Vegetables: 5 servings.

▶ At least 2 litres (4 pints) of water, tea, coffee or other sugar-free or low-calorie drinks.

If you wish, you can also include:

▶ Sugar-free chewing gum or liquorice root (available from health food shops).

▶ Up to 10 sugar-free mints.

Protein foods

You can eat generous amounts of the following protein foods on your two restricted days of The 2-Day Diet:

▶ For women: a minimum of 4 servings and a maximum of 12 servings from the list below per day.

▶ For men: a minimum of 4 servings and a maximum of 14 servings from the list below per day.

You can have any number of protein servings in a meal but make sure you keep within the maximum daily allowances.

Protein	1 serving[†] equal to:
Fresh or smoked* white fish (for example, haddock or cod)	60 g (2 oz) (two fish-finger sized pieces)
Tinned tuna in brine or spring water	45 g (1½ oz)
Oily fish (fresh or tinned) in tomato sauce or oil (drained), for example, mackerel, sardines, salmon, trout, tuna, smoked salmon* or trout* or kippers*	30 g (1 oz)
Seafood, e.g. prawns, mussels, crab	45 g (1½ oz)
Chicken, turkey or duck (cooked without the skin)	30 g (1 oz) (a slice the size of a playing card)
Lean beef, pork, lamb, rabbit, venison or offal (fat removed)	30 g (1 oz) per serving to a maximum of 500 g (1 lb 1 oz) per week for women and 600 g (1 lb 4 oz) per week for men (including the two restricted days and five unrestricted days of The 2-Day Diet)
Lean bacon*	1 grilled rasher
Lean ham*	2 medium or 4 wafer-thin slices
Eggs	1 medium/large egg
Tofu	50 g (1¾ oz)

*see page 55   †weights are given for uncooked meat and fish. Cooked meats will weigh about one third less than uncooked.

how to do the two restricted days

You can only include one of the following protein foods on each restricted day as they contain some carbohydrate. They count towards your daily protein allowance.

Protein	Maximum	Servings
Textured vegetable protein (TVP)	maximum 30 g (1 oz) per day	3
Soya and edamame beans	60 g (2 oz) per day	2
Low-fat hummus	maximum 1 heaped tablespoon (30 g/1 oz) per day	1
Quorn	maximum 115 g (4 oz) per day	4

What you need to know about protein

Protein is a key part of your two restricted days on The 2-Day Diet as well as the rest of the week, because it is the most filling food you can eat. In fact, research suggests that our appetites are fundamentally controlled by our need for protein and the body will keep telling you that you are hungry until you have eaten enough of it. If you eat a diet that's low in protein, you need to consume a lot of calories before you reach this point – which may be one reason why so many people overeat, especially dieters striving to keep to one of the numerous low-protein, low-fat weight-loss diet plans. Protein is also vital for maintaining muscle mass when you diet. Dieters who have successfully lost weight seem to be more likely to overeat and regain the weight they have lost if they have lost a lot of muscle as well as fat when they lost weight. This is a 'feedback', which is the body's way of trying to replace the muscle lost through dieting. Protein foods are also helpful to dieters because they burn an extra 65–70 calories to absorb and digest them.

Fats

You can have generous amounts of the following foods:

▶ For women: a maximum of 5 servings from the list below per day.

▶ For men: a maximum of 6 servings per day.

Fat	1 serving equal to:
Margarine or low-fat spread (avoid the 'buttery' types)	1 teaspoon (8 g)
Olive oil or other oil (not palm, coconut or ghee)	1 dessertspoon (7 g)
Oil-based dressing	1 dessertspoon (7 g)
Unsalted or salted* or dry roasted nuts (not honey roast).	1 dessertspoon or 3 walnut halves, 3 Brazil nuts, 4 almonds, 8 peanuts, 10 cashews or 10 pistachios (not chestnuts)
Pesto	1 teaspoon (8 g)
Mayonnaise	1 teaspoon (5 g)
Low-fat mayonnaise	1 tablespoon (15 g)
Olives*	10
Peanut butter (without palm oil)	1 teaspoon (8 g)

* see page 55

You can only have one of the following fatty foods on each restricted day as they contain some carbohydrate. They count towards your fat serving allowance.

Fat	Maximum	Servings
Avocado	½ pear	2
Guacamole	2 tablespoons	2
Low-fat Guacamole	2 tablespoons	1

Dairy foods

Choose up to three servings from the following list per day:

Dairy	1 serving equal to:
Milk (semi-skimmed or skimmed)	200 ml (⅓ pint/7 fl oz)
Soya milk (sweetened or unsweetened with added calcium)†	200 ml (⅓ pint/7 fl oz)
Yoghurt: diet fruit, plain soya; Greek, plain or fromage frais (all low fat)	1 small pot 120–150 g (4–5 oz) or 3 heaped tablespoons
Whole milk plain yoghurt	80–90 g (2½–3 oz) or 2 heaped tablespoons
Cottage cheese	75 g (2½ oz) or 2 tablespoons
Quark	⅓ pot or 3 tablespoons (90 g/3 oz)
Cream cheese (light or extra-light)	1 tablespoon (30 g/1 oz)
Lower-fat cheeses: reduced-fat Cheddar, Edam, Bavarian smoked, feta*, Camembert, ricotta, mozzarella, reduced-fat halloumi	Matchbox size – 30 g (1 oz) per serving to a maximum of 120 g (4 oz) for women per week and 150 g (5 oz) for men on restricted and un-restricted days

† Don't be tempted to use rice or oat milk instead of dairy or soya milk. They are unsuitable for restricted days as they are too low in protein and too high in carbohydrates. However, you can use them on the five unrestricted days.

*see page 55

'Strangely for me I didn't have cravings for chocolate or biscuits on my two restricted days, but I did long for bread, cereals and other not-so-naughty food experiences.'
Val, 43

Fruit

You can include one piece of fruit, but only the lower-carbohydrate fruits from the list below. If you prefer you can have an extra vegetable serving instead of fruit. You can sweeten fruit with artificial sweeteners, as required, but do not add sugar.

Fruit	1 serving equal to 80 g (2½ oz)
Apricots	3 fresh or dried
Blackberries	1 handful
Blackcurrants	4 heaped tablespoons
Redcurrants	4 heaped tablespoons
Grapefruit, guava	½ whole fruit
Melon	5 cm (2 in) slice
Pineapple	1 large slice
Peach	1 fruit
Papaya	1 slice
Passion fruit	5 fruits
Raspberries	2 handfuls
Strawberries	7
Stewed rhubarb, gooseberries or cranberries	3 heaped tablespoons with sweetener

'It was easier than I expected and it's got easier as time has gone on. I soon got into the habit of eating less on the restricted days and have become used to eating less. I think it also helped to eat the same kind of food over the two days, making serving sizes easy to follow.' Lyndsey, 35

'The 2-Day Diet makes me feel good because it gives me control and focus for two days of the week.' Carol, 39

Vegetables

Only the following lower-carbohydrate vegetables are allowed.
Choose five servings of vegetables per day from the list below.

Vegetables	1 serving equal to 80 g (2½ oz)
Artichoke	2 globe hearts
Asparagus, tinned	7 spears
Asparagus, fresh	5 spears
Aubergine	⅓ medium
Beans, French	4 heaped tablespoons
Beans, runner	4 heaped tablespoons
Beansprouts, fresh	2 handfuls
Broccoli	2 spears
Brussels sprouts	8
Cabbage	⅙ small cabbage or 3 heaped tablespoons shredded leaves
Cauliflower	8 florets
Celeriac	3 heaped tablespoons
Celery	3 sticks
Chinese leaves	⅕ 'head'
Courgette	½ large courgette
Cucumber	5 cm (2 in) piece
Curly kale, cooked	4 heaped tablespoons
Fennel	½ cup sliced
Karela or gourd	½
Leeks	1 medium
Lettuce (mixed leaves) or rocket	1 cereal bowlful

Vegetables	1 serving equal to 80 g (2½ oz)
Mangetout	1 handful
Mushrooms, fresh	14 button or 3 handfuls of slices
Mushrooms, dried	2 tablespoons or handful porcini
Okra	16 medium
Pak choi (Chinese cabbage)	2 handfuls
Pepper (green only)	½
Pumpkin	3 heaped tablespoons
Radish	10
Spinach, cooked	2 heaped tablespoons
Spinach, fresh	1 cereal bowlful
Spring greens, cooked	4 heaped tablespoons
Spring onion	8
Sweetcorn, baby (whole not kernels)	6
Tomato, tinned	2 plum tomatoes or ½ tin chopped
Tomato, fresh	1 medium or 7 cherry
Tomato purée	1 heaped tablespoon
Tomato, sundried	4 pieces
Watercress	1 cereal bowlful

Flavourings

You can use these flavourings freely:

▶ Lemon juice

▶ Fresh or dried herbs and spices

▶ Black pepper

▶ Mustard/horseradish

- Vinegars, e.g. red or white wine vinegar, balsamic vinegar or rice wine vinegar

- Fresh or pre-chopped garlic or ginger

- Chilli – fresh, powdered or dried flakes

- Soy sauce/low-salt soy sauce (look for varieties with added

- chilli for an extra kick!)*

- Miso paste

- Fish sauce*

- Worcester sauce*

Salt

Because you will be fat-burning on your restricted days and passing water and electrolytes from your body, it's important to ensure that you take in some salt. You don't need huge amounts: include up to 5–6 g salt on those days (the equivalent to 2,000–2,400 mg sodium).

If you find that you are developing headaches on your restricted days this may indicate that you need a little more salt.

There is some salt naturally occurring in some of the foods you will eat – for example: dairy foods, fish and seafood. If you wish you can include 4–6 servings of foods that are higher in salt on your restricted days. These foods are indicated in the food lists above with *.

Alternatively you can include one of the following:

- ½ stock cube or 2 teaspoons bouillon as a drink or in food.

- 1 tablespoon soy sauce.

- 1 teaspoon yeast extract or meat stock with hot water.

- 3 teaspoons gravy powder or granules dissolved in hot water.

Do not include a salty drink or salty foods if you are taking a water tablet for high blood pressure.

Since too much salt is bad for blood pressure and bones we recommend you limit these salty foods during the rest of the week to just one serving per week (see page 72).

> *'I have found this diet really easy to follow. I can still eat a wide variety of foods and I love that I only need to wait a day or two if I have a serious chocolate or cake craving. Even better, I don't feel guilty about it when I do treat myself. I plan my two diet days around my social life, so it doesn't interfere at all. I plan my two days carefully to eat foods that will sustain me and keep me going, while giving me the nutrients I need. I do feel healthier and lighter on my toes!'*
> Andrea, 30

Ideas for low-calorie drinks

It is very important to drink plenty on your two restricted days of The 2-Day Diet. Aim to drink 2 litres (4 pints) from this list to prevent dehydration, constipation and headaches, and to help keep hunger pangs at bay:

▶ Water (still or sparkling).

▶ Tea and coffee (black or add milk as required from your daily milk allowance, use sweeteners as required).

▶ Flavoured sugar-free sparkling water – make sure you check the label and avoid brands containing added sugar.

▶ Sugar-free or no-added-sugar fruit-flavoured squash made up with still or sparkling water. Avoid 'high juice' varieties because they contain natural fruit sugars; instead, choose no-added-sugar varieties sweetened with artificial sweeteners.

▶ Fruit, herbal or green teas.

▶ Diet, sugar-free or no-added-sugar fizzy drinks (up to 3 litres/6 pints per week – see page 86).

▶ Grated ginger in boiling water (and sweeteners as required). Drink hot or allow to cool first, then chill.

▶ Slice of lemon or lime in boiling water.

You can sweeten all drinks with artificial sweeteners as required. Do not add sugar (see page 73). See The 2-Day Diet recipe chapter (see page 180) for some refreshing drinks you can make.

The vegetarian 2-Day Diet

If you are vegetarian you can easily follow The 2-Day Diet. The vegetarian version is similar, but as some vegetarian sources of protein contain carbohydrates you will need to eat slightly less of the dairy foods since these also contain carbohydrates. Your selection of protein foods is more limited than for meat- and fish-eaters, but it is extremely important to include the recommended amounts of protein and low-fat dairy foods to make sure you don't get hungry. The recipe section (see page 180) is packed with many interesting meals you can prepare with eggs, tofu, soya beans and textured vegetable protein (TVP).

Protein foods

▶ For women: a minimum of 4 servings and a maximum of 12 servings from the list below per day.

▶ For men: a minimum of 4 servings and a maximum of 14 servings from the list below per day.

On your two restricted days of The 2-Day Diet you can have generous amounts of eggs and tofu within your daily allowance:

Protein	1 serving equal to:
Eggs	1 medium/large egg
Tofu	50 g (1¾ oz)

You can also choose up to six protein servings from the following list each day. Make sure that you get no more than 15 g per day of total carbohydrates from this section.

Protein	1 serving equal to:
Vegetarian sausage/burger with < 5 g carb	½
Textured vegetable protein, uncooked	2 teaspoons (10 g/⅓oz)
Soya beans (frozen or cooked)	2 tablespoons (30 g/1 oz)
Low-fat hummus	1 heaped tablespoon (30 g/1 oz)
Tempeh	40 g (1½ oz)
Quorn mince/pieces or fillet	30 g (1 oz)
Edamame beans (frozen or cooked)	2 tablespoons (30 g/1 oz)

NB: Avoid burgers and fillets with a breadcrumb coating as these will be higher in carbohydrate.

A word about eggs

Eggs have had a bad press, but contrary to popular belief they are a great diet food that you can eat freely. They're high in protein, low in fat, contain only 70 calories a serving and are a great source of vitamins A and D (an egg can provide 10 per cent of your daily requirement of vitamin D), selenium, calcium, iron, zinc and folate.

Although many people worry that eggs are high in cholesterol, they are not linked to heart disease and a recent study found that people on a low-fat diet who ate two eggs each day lost weight, with no adverse effects on their cholesterol levels. In fact, their levels of the beneficial form of cholesterol in the body, the 'HDL cholesterol', actually increased.[1]

Dairy foods

You can have up to 60 g (2 oz) of lower-fat cheese, but no more than 120 g (4 oz) per week for women and 150 g (5 oz) for men, including the two restricted and five un-restricted days, such as:

▶ Reduced-fat Cheddar

▶ Feta

▶ Mozzarella

▶ Bavarian smoked cheese

▶ Camembert

▶ Edam

▶ Ricotta

▶ Reduced-fat Halloumi

You can also choose two servings from the following list per day:

Dairy	1 serving equal to:
Milk (semi-skimmed or skimmed)	200 ml (⅓ pint/7 fl oz)
Soya milk (sweetened or unsweetened with added calcium)†	200 ml (⅓ pint/7 fl oz)

Dairy	1 serving equal to:
Yoghurt: diet fruit, plain soya; Greek, fromage frais (all low fat)	1 small pot 120–150 g (4–5 oz) or plain or 3 heaped tablespoons
Whole milk plain yoghurt tablespoons	80–90 g (2½–3 oz) or 2 heaped
Cottage cheese	75 g (2½ oz) or 2 tablespoons
Quark	⅓ pot or 3 tablespoons (90 g/3 oz)
Cream cheese (light or extra-light)	1 tablespoon (30 g/1 oz)

† Don't be tempted to use rice or oat milk instead of dairy or soya milk. They are unsuitable for restricted days as they are too low in protein and too high in carbohydrates. However, you can use them on the other five unrestricted days.

Make sure that you include the allowance of fat, vegetables and fruit on your restricted days (see pages 50–57).

Your questions answered

'Do I need to take a vitamin supplement on the two restricted days of The 2-Day Diet?'

You don't need to take a supplement on The 2-Day Diet. When you go on any weight-loss diet and eat less you often reduce your intake of vitamins and minerals. It's always better to get the nutrients you need from food as this ensures a gradual supply of nutrients that are more easily absorbed by your body. The one-off dose delivered in a supplement can lead to fluxes of abnormally high levels, which may not be good for your body. For example, there is currently a concern that high-dose calcium supplements cause high blood levels of calcium; which can lead to calcification and damage to the arteries and possibly heart disease. The 2-Day Diet is designed to ensure that you get the nutrients you need. The nutrients that your diet may be lacking on the two restricted days of The 2-Day Diet are calcium, iron, zinc and magnesium and we find that many people, including our Dieters, will already have low intakes of selenium, folate and vitamin A in their normal diet. Good sources of these important nutrients on your restricted days are:

▶ Calcium from low-fat dairy foods, calcium-fortified soya milk, tinned oily fish if you eat the bones, tofu set with calcium, almonds, eggs and green, leafy vegetables.

▶ Iron from lean meat, eggs, nuts and green vegetables.

▶ Zinc from lean meat, milk, eggs, nuts and cheese.

▶ Magnesium from lean meat, poultry, fish, Quorn, nuts, soya beans and green vegetables.

▶ Selenium from meat, fish, Brazil nuts and eggs.

▶ Folate from asparagus and green, leafy vegetables.

▶ Vitamin A from eggs, cheese and margarines.

It is also important to include good dietary sources of these foods on unrestricted days too. For a full guide to good nutrient sources on the two restricted and five unrestricted days of The 2-Day Diet see www.thetwodaydiet.co.uk.

'Should I be eating lots of nuts – aren't they very high in calories?'

Many of our 2-Day Dieters worry about eating nuts because they are high in fat and therefore calories. However, they are packed with healthy monounsaturated and omega-3 fats (see page 75) and because they are high in protein they are also very filling. They may even help reduce the risk of heart disease because they contain arginine, a substance that may make your artery walls more flexible and less prone to blood clots. Eat unsalted varieties of nuts to keep your salt intake down, unless you are using them as a salty food on the restricted days of The 2-Day Diet (see page 55).

'How easy is The 2-Day Diet to follow?'

Many of our 2-Day Dieters were surprised by how easy they found The 2-Day Diet. Because it is simple but structured they quickly adapted to it and got into a routine. Only 3 per cent of our 2-Day Dieters reported having problems fitting it into their daily lives and with family meals. You will need to plan ahead, but because you are only dieting for two days, making larger quantities and freezing them will give you a good range of different meals to choose from. Many of our 2-Day Dieters found that the 2-Day Diet actually became easier the longer they were on it. As one woman said, 'Unlike other diets, which are okay at first and get harder over time, I found The 2-Day Diet quite hard to begin with, but it got easier the more your body and mind got used to what you were doing.'

'Will I be hungry on my diet days?'

You should not feel any hungrier on your two restricted days of The 2-Day Diet than you do normally. We assessed 'hungriness' in our 2-Day Dieters before starting the Diet and while they were doing it using hunger scales. We found that they scored their 'hungriness' exactly the same on their restricted and un-restricted days as they had before they started The 2-Day Diet. It can be easy to mistake hunger for thirst, so if you feel hungry, try having a drink and see if that helps. On the two restricted days of The 2-Day Diet make sure that you have enough protein foods, nuts, dairy foods and vegetables, which are particularly good at filling you up. If you do feel hungry the first few times you try the Diet, stick with it, as most of our 2-Day Dieters found that it got easier as they got used to it.

Snack ideas for the two restricted days of The 2-Day Diet

- Olives.
- Handful of nuts (not chestnuts).
- Fruit from the allowed list.
- Vegetable crudités, such as celery, cucumber, green peppers, mange tout, spring onion and cherry tomatoes, with salsa, low-fat hummus, tuna pâté, tsatsiki or guacamole (see pages 196, 194 and 195).
- Plain or diet yoghurt.
- Bowl of soup (see page 187).
- Salad or cooked vegetables with cottage cheese, low-fat cream cheese or hummus.
- Half a pot of cottage cheese.
- Smoothie made with yoghurt, skimmed or semi-skimmed milk and one piece of fruit.
- Half a tin of sardines or pilchards.
- Salty drink (see page 55).
- Sautéed tofu or chicken strips lightly fried in spices.
- Boiled egg.
- Avocado, mozzarella, tomato and basil skewers or stacks.
- Celery sticks filled with low-fat cream cheese.
- Asparagus spears dipped in egg.
- Sugar-free jelly.
- Ice lolly made from frozen, diluted, sugar-free squash.

'Will the 2-Day Diet help me to permanently change my eating habits?'

The two restricted days of The 2-Day Diet helped our Dieters recognise their habitual 'unhealthy' eating habits and behaviours. The two restricted days helped them to practise and get into the habit of eating healthier foods and smaller servings each week. On top of that they began to recognise, often for the first time in a long time, what was 'real' hunger or thirst, rather than just wanting to eat for the sake of it. They learnt to really enjoy and savour their food on both the two restricted and five unrestricted days. The 2-Day Diet helps put you back in control of your eating.

'Why am I passing more water?'

One thing you will notice on your restricted days is that you will be going to the toilet more often. This is for two reasons: firstly, because you will be mobilising glycogen, the carbohydrate stored in your muscles and liver; this releases water into the body that the body then needs to get rid of; secondly, burning fat also increases the levels of ketones in the blood which acts as a diuretic (in the same way as tea and coffee), making you want to pass more water.

Ketones are a natural by-product of burning fat in the body. They are not thought to have harmful effects unless they build up to extremely high levels, which won't happen on The 2-Day Diet. Ketones have a bad press as the levels achieved with some daily, very low-carbohydrate diets can lead to side effects such as headaches, nausea or bad breath. Our Dieters typically doubled their level of ketones, in contrast to dieters on longer-term, low-carbohydrate diets who experience five-fold increases in ketones.

'Will I feel more tired on my diet days?'

Quite the contrary! Most of our 2-Day Dieters were very positive about the way they felt while doing the Diet. Many said they felt invigorated, cleansed and detoxed during and after the two restricted days each week. This made them more committed and motivated to keep to The 2-Day Diet each week and, importantly, to eat healthily for the rest of the week. They reported feeling less bloated after eating, less sluggish and more energetic and when we assessed their general mood and well-being, we found that their scores for tension, depression, anger, fatigue and confusion were halved, while in nearly all cases their mood improved.

Interestingly, our 2-Day Dieters said that the two restricted days each week gave them all the positive feelings that dieters often experience during the first few days of following a normal diet, with the positive feelings of increased energy and sense of achievement that go with it. Revisiting those feelings every week gave them a real boost and reinforced their motivation to succeed.

'Are there any side effects?'

None of our 2-Day Dieters reported major problems, although a few experienced headaches. If this happens, make sure you are drinking plenty (2 litres/4 pints a day is usually enough). You can drink more than this, but you will need to ensure you are including enough electrolytes as well, i.e. potassium, sodium (salt) and also magnesium, which you will get by eating your recommended servings of fruit, vegetables, dairy and protein foods. You may find you need to include a salty food or drink on the two restricted days of The 2-Day Diet (see page 55). Although it's not necessary to cut down on tea and coffee on the Diet, if you find you are drinking less of these than usual since starting it, your headaches may be related to caffeine withdrawal. The drop in carbohydrate intake on the two days can also cause headaches, but this should improve as your body gets used to it.

A few 2-Day Dieters found they became constipated. If this happens make sure you are getting enough fluid and having your full fruit and vegetable allowance on restricted days. On your unrestricted days make sure you eat plenty of fibre by having your full allowance of fruit and vegetables, choosing carbohydrates that are high in fibre (see page 336) drinking plenty, and meeting the recommendations for exercise.

'I'm worried that I won't be able to concentrate at work on my restricted days'

A few Dieters – again only 3 per cent – found concentration difficult, although it is possible that they were expecting problems and so any effects were exaggerated. There's no consistent evidence that either low-calorie or low-carbohydrate diets affect concentration. In one recent study in the USA students were given either a very low-calorie drink (150 kcal, 30 g carbohydrates) or a drink that contained their full calorie requirement (2,300 kcal, 560 g carbohydrate) per day for two days without being told which drink they were getting. None receiving the low-calorie drink reported any problems with concentration, energy levels or mood[2]. Other research suggests that low-carb, high-protein diets could actually increase memory and alertness[3] and have been used to treat older adults with cognitive impairment[4].

If you genuinely feel that you are struggling to concentrate or feel lightheaded:

▶ Make sure you are well hydrated and are getting enough salt (sodium) (see page 55), potassium and magnesium by

including recommended foods. See the nutrient list at
www.thetwodaydiet.co.uk.

▶ Make sure that you are getting the 50 g of carbohydrates
allowed on restricted days (found in your dairy and fruit and
vegetable allowances).

'Will my breath smell on The 2-Day Diet?'

A few of our Dieters complained about having a bad taste
in their mouth, but this was usually minor and not enough
to make their breath smell. The taste is caused by ketones,
substances that build up when your body burns fat to use for
energy. Although you may notice it on the two restricted days,
it will disappear on the other five unrestricted days. Drinking
more may help and you can also suck sugar-free mints (up to
10 a day).

'Aren't the two days of The 2-Day Diet just the same as an Atkins or Dukan-style diet?'

The two restricted days of The 2-Day Diet are low-carb and so
have some similarities to low-carb, high-protein diets such as
Atkins or Dukan, but this diet is different. The low-carb days
of The 2-Day Diet are designed for weight loss and are also
designed for optimum health, ensuring that you get the right
balance of healthy fats (low in saturates, high in monounsatur-
ates and omega-3 fats), and fruit and vegetables. Remember,
you are only eating low carb for two days of the week. When
you combine the two days with a healthy balanced Mediterranean diet for the rest of the week it makes The 2-Day Diet
very different from other diets.

'How much will the diet cost – will my food bill go up?'

The 2-Day Diet should cost you less than you are spending now. Before they started dieting our Dieters spent, on average, £42 on food and drink for themselves each week. This included £36 on food and nearly £6 on alcohol. Of the money spent on food nearly £6 was spent on ready meals, £4.50 on takeaways, and an average of £3 on sweets, cakes and biscuits. On The 2-Day Diet their total food bill dropped by £9 per week. They were now spending £33 a week on food and drink because they had cut back on ready meals, alcohol and sweet foods. You can either pocket the difference or set it aside to treat yourself when you reach your diet goals. One important change was that the amount they spent per calorie did increase with the higher nutritional quality of their diet – this rose from just under 2p per calorie to 2.5p per calorie. However, because they were eating fewer calories their overall food bill was lower. The recipes and meal ideas in this book (see pages 170–312) include plenty of healthy and reasonably priced options, so being on The 2-Day Diet does not mean that you have to spend more on food.

Summary

▶ For the two restricted days of The 2-Day Diet you are limited to eating protein, fats, five servings of low-carb vegetables, one serving of fruit and some low-fat dairy foods. It's important to stick to the restricted foods, not exceed the maximum number of servings allowed, and get enough protein, which will help to keep you full and maintain muscle in your body.

▶ No high-carbohydrate foods such as bread, cake, sweets or alcohol are allowed on the two restricted days.

▶ You don't need to take any supplements as The 2-Day Diet is balanced to meet all your nutritional needs.

▶ To get the full benefits of the Diet do your two restricted days together (one after the other).

▶ The majority of Dieters find the two restricted days of The 2-Day Diet are easy to adapt to and fit into their lifestyle.

▶ Most Dieters don't feel hungry. Instead they feel healthier and have more energy while doing the Diet. A small minority may experience minor side effects, which are easily remedied.

4

how to eat
on the five
unrestricted days

Your diet for the remaining days (the five unrestricted days) on The 2-Day Diet should be based on eating a healthy Mediterranean-style diet. This includes food that is as whole and unprocessed as possible, with lots of fruit and veget- ables, wholegrains, beans, pulses, nuts and olive oil as well as fish, poultry, low-fat dairy foods, and it can include small amounts of lean, red meat – but not lots of pasta, pizza and red wine!

The Mediterranean diet

The Mediterranean diet is packed full of disease-fighting anti-oxidants, vitamins and flavonoids and the benefits of eating this way are almost too numerous to list. There's convincing evidence that it not only lowers the risk of heart disease and type 2 diabetes, but it may also protect against some cancers and Alzheimer's disease[1]. Your eating plan for these five unrestricted days contains high-protein, high-fibre foods to help you feel full and reduce your chances of overeating. Don't be tempted to overeat or eat junk food on these five unrestricted days – follow the guidelines below to give yourself the best possible chance of successful weight loss. A full guide to recommended servings for the unrestricted days can be found in Appendix C (see pages 322–327).

Protein foods

Include:

▶ White or oily fish and seafood.

▶ Chicken, turkey or duck (cooked without skin).

▶ Lean cuts of red meat – for example beef, pork, lamb or offal, lean game, venison, rabbit or pheasant (maximum 500 g/1 lb 1 oz a week for women and 600 g/1 lb 4 oz a week for men, including the two restricted and five unrestricted days of The 2-Day Diet).

▶ Pulses, beans, chickpeas and lentils – use these for bulking up dishes.

Limit to once during the five unrestricted days

▶ Fatty cuts of red meat, poultry and game (these are high in saturated fat).

▶ High-fat processed meat and meat products (for example sausage and corned beef – these are high in saturated fat and salt).

▶ Charred and well-done meat and fish (these are limited

due to some concerns about cancer risk associated with consuming charred foods).

▶ Battered/breaded fish (these are higher in calories and much lower in protein than uncoated fish).

▶ Low-fat processed meats, bacon, ham and salty fish such as kippers, smoked salmon, smoked mackerel and smoked white fish to limit your overall salt intake for the week.

You can include salty foods on your two restricted days as you may be losing fluid and salt from the body (see page 55).

All about carbs

Carbohydrates provide most of our energy – typically 50 to 60 per cent of our calories. Contrary to popular belief, a traditional Mediterranean diet is not based on foods such as pasta and pizza but actually contains less than 45 per cent of your calories as carbohydrates. Because your two restricted days contain very few carbohydrates, your overall 2-Day Diet for the week has around 40 per cent of its energy from carbohydrates – more in line with our hunter-gatherer ancestors, who are thought to have obtained between 20 and 40 per cent of their calories from carbohydrates.

When it comes to carbohydrates, choose wholegrain varieties whenever possible. They contain more fibre and nutrients than processed or white versions, take longer to digest and absorb, and can keep you feeling full for longer. Cut down on white, refined carbohydrates and sugar and try to avoid sugary snacks such as sweets and cakes. These carbohydrates are quickly digested and lead to spikes in blood sugar and high levels of insulin, which in turn increase your appetite and leave you craving more!

Sugar provides four calories per gram, but has no other nutrients, which is why it is often referred to as 'empty' calories. Too much of any kind of sugar is bad for you, but be particularly wary of foods containing added fructose (often labelled as 'high fructose corn syrup' or 'glucose fructose syrup') found in some breakfast cereals, cereal bars, sweetened fruit juices or high-juice squash, yoghurts, rice puddings, fromage frais, biscuits, cakes and ice cream.

There is growing concern about the damaging effects of fructose, both because of its high-calorie content and because it is directly converted to fat that builds up in the liver. A fatty liver is less able to remove fat circulating in the blood (see page 42) so this fat is deposited in the blood vessels, leading to narrowing of the vessels and raised blood pressure. In a recent study, people who ate an extra 1,000 calories in sweets and sugary drinks for three weeks showed an alarming three-fold increase in the amount of fat in their livers. This was reversed when they subsequently followed a low-calorie Mediterranean diet[2].

Fructose is also found naturally in fruit in far smaller amounts than in processed foods: an apple, for example, only contains one-fifth of the fructose of a regular can of cola. Fructose in fruit does not seem to have any adverse effects on health as fruit also contains protective plant polyphenols. One of the reasons for the harmful effects of the modern Western diet is the large amounts of refined carbohydrates listed in the left-hand column of the table overleaf.

Switch from these carbs ...	... to these
White bread, French stick, bagels, croissants, crumpets	Granary bread, pitta bread, pumpernickel bread, multigrain bread, rye bread, wholemeal bread
White rice, couscous, noodles	Basmati rice, bulgur wheat, quinoa, brown rice, brown noodles, wholewheat pasta, brown couscous, brown rice
Cornflakes, white rice cereal, sugary cereals, instant oat cereal	Porridge, bran flakes, high-fibre bran cereal, wholewheat bisks, no-added-sugar muesli
Crisps, sweets, biscuits, sugary popcorn, doughnuts, cakes	Yoghurts, nuts, plain popcorn
Mashed potato, chips	Sweet potatoes, new potatoes boiled in their skins, jacket potatoes
Cream crackers, rice cakes	Oatcakes, rye crispbreads, wholewheat crackers
Sugary, fizzy drinks	Water, sugar-free squash, diet fizzy drinks

*'The diet is easy as long as you are organised.
I haven't felt the need for chocolate, crisps etc.
This is dieting without feeling hungry and losing weight
without feeling deprived.'* Chris, 63

Your 'five a day'

We need fruit and vegetables to protect us from heart disease and strokes, to help control blood pressure and keep our bones healthy. Fruit and vegetables may also help protect against certain cancers, although the links with cancer are not as strong or compelling as they are for heart disease[3]. Fruit and vegetables may also reduce the risk of dementia.

On the two restricted days of The 2-Day Diet you are allowed to have five servings of lower-carbohydrate vegetables and one low-carbohydrate fruit, but for the five unrestricted days of the rest of the week you can include a variety of fruits and vegetables (including higher-carbohydrate ones). You should aim to have two servings of fruit and five servings of vegetables per day. Don't assume that eating fruit and vegetables will mean that you will naturally want to eat less of other foods. In fact, when researchers asked overweight people to include six to eight servings of fruit and vegetables a day in their diet many just added this to what they normally ate and gained 4½ lb (2 kg) over the eight weeks of the study[4].

We recommend eating more vegetables than fruit as they usually provide fewer calories – for example a banana can contain between 80 and 160 calories, depending on size, while 20 mushrooms contain only 16 calories and a large serving of broccoli only 12 calories. Vegetables are a great way to fill up your plate while adding very few calories. As a dieter you may already know that a small bar of chocolate provides 300 calories. For the same number of calories you could eat a whopping 1 kg (2 lb) of broccoli!

'It's so great to be losing weight and knowing that I'm eating healthily. I love the fish, chicken and salads on the Mediterranean days.' Anna, 43

Fat facts

We all need some fat in our diet, but too much leads to us piling on the pounds (a gram of carbohydrate contains four calories, whereas a gram of fat contains nine). Therefore try not to add extra fat when you are cooking and opt for grilling, microwaving or steaming when you can and if you do use oil, just use a little olive, soy or rapeseed oil, or a few squirts of spray oil.

Cut down on saturated fats, since these are the harmful fats that clog arteries. Saturated fats are found in fatty red meat, processed meats and sausages, full-fat dairy products, palm oil, chocolate and coconut oil. Try to replace them with 'healthy' fats, especially monounsaturated fats in olives, olive oil, rapeseed oil, avocados, nuts (such as peanuts, almonds, pecans, hazelnuts, cashews and pistachios), which can help to lower cholesterol levels.

Omega-3 fats have important roles for health as they help to maintain a healthy heart, lower blood pressure and blood fat levels. They also have anti-inflammatory effects, which help to maintain a healthy brain and nervous system, and reduce the risk of diabetes and certain cancers. The body also needs omega-6 fats; however, the modern diet contains too few omega-3 fats and an excess of omega-6, which results in omega-3 fats not being able to carry out their good work.

The best way to redress the balance is to consume more omega-3, found in oily fish such as salmon, sardines, mackerel and fresh tuna (not tinned) and for vegetarians omega-3-enriched eggs, flaxseed, walnuts and rapeseed oil. Don't overdo omega-6-rich foods such as corn, sunflower oil, turkey and game meat, shellfish, tinned tuna, pine nuts and sesame seeds.

'I've always found diets difficult before – as life tends to get in the way. The 2-Day Diet's been so much easier as you can work it around whatever else is going on. You can go to parties, weddings, meals out and still lose weight!'
Mary, 31

Make sure you drink enough

Most of us don't drink anywhere near enough, and it's especially important to stay well hydrated when you are trying to lose weight. We recommend at least eight glasses of fluid each day

(2 litres/4 pints) to help you feel full, keep you hydrated and to prevent constipation. We often mistake thirst for hunger, so if you fancy something to eat, have a drink first and see if your cravings go away. In fact, some research suggests that drinking water before you eat could help you eat less at mealtimes – and drinking cold water may actually boost your metabolic rate for up to an hour after drinking[5]. However, don't get too excited! It will only burn five extra calories a day, but this can add up over the year – and every little helps. Some people worry about drinking too much and there have been occasional reports of excessive water intake (more than 5 litres/10 pints per day) leading to water toxicity, with dilution of the salts in the blood. This is only really a problem if large volumes of water are drunk over a short time; you should ideally drink no more than 1 litre (2 pints) over an hour.

Normal, non-diet fizzy drinks are a major problem in our Western diet. They are packed with sugars (about 10 teaspoons per can), contain around 150 calories, but contain no nutrients and are quickly converted to fat in the body.

What to drink

You need to have at least 8 drinks or 2 litres (4 pints) a day:

▶ Water (still or sparkling).

▶ Tea – black or green, caffeinated or decaffeinated.

▶ Coffee – caffeinated or decaffeinated.

▶ Herbal and fruit teas.

▶ Sugar-free or diet squash or fizzy drinks (less than 3 litres/6 pints per week – see page 86).

Limit the following

▶ Alcohol.

▶ Adding sugar to drinks.

▶ Non-diet fizzy drinks.

▶ Fruit juice (a maximum of 200 ml/7 fl oz per day).

▶ Vegetable juice (a maximum of 200 ml/7 fl oz per day).

Fruit juice

People assume that a glass of pure, unsweetened fruit juice is a healthy addition to your meal. By all means have a glass a day, but it's always better to eat a piece of whole fruit instead. Not only is fruit juice high in calories, but it contains no fibre and won't be as filling as eating a piece of fruit. In one study people were given either an apple or some apple juice, and were then asked to eat a meal until they were full. The apple-eaters ate less at the meal and 15 per cent fewer calories overall than those given juice to drink[6].

Why fibre is important for our health and weight

Fibre is found in the plant foods we eat and is vital for anyone who is trying to lose weight and follow the 2-Day Diet. Fibre helps you feel full for longer, keeps your blood sugar stable and keeps your bowel functioning optimally. There are two main types of fibre, both of which are important for the Dieter.

Insoluble fibre

This is found in cereals and pulses. It protects against constipation and helps keep your bowel healthy by preventing the build-up of toxic substances (the by-products of digested protein), which have been linked to bowel cancer. Since The 2-Day Diet includes plenty of protein, it is really important to make sure you have enough of this type of fibre on unrestricted days.

Soluble fibre
Found in oats, barley, beans, fruit and vegetables, soluble fibre slows down the rate at which food empties from your stomach.

Why fibre is vital for your health

Fibre plays a key role in maintaining the balance of beneficial bacteria in your gut. Each of us has about 100 trillion bacteria in our bowels (weighing around 4 lb/1.8 kg). Their number gives an indication of their importance to our health. Recent studies indicate that there are healthy combinations of bacteria, which if disrupted by poor diet, can actually lead to diseases and even obesity. Bacteria ferment the fibre we eat and produce fats known as 'short chain' fats. A growing body of research indicates that eating plenty of fibre results in the right bacteria in the bowel which then produce the right fats. These have three key roles in protecting our health:

- The fats are an essential fuel for the cells lining the bowel, and keep these cells healthy.
- Some of the fats produced in the bowel are absorbed, circulate in the bloodstream and reduce sugar levels and the levels of disease-producing fats in the blood.
- Having the right bacteria in the gut may also affect your weight. Overweight people have a different balance of gut bacteria, which can cause weight gain[7].

It also slows down the absorption of nutrients, avoiding surges in blood sugar after meals and helping to keep blood sugar stable. Soluble fibre helps to lower cholesterol too.

Make sure you include your permitted fruit and vegetables on the two restricted days of The 2-Day Diet. Aim to have at least 24 g of fibre a day on your unrestricted days, with a good mix of soluble and insoluble types (see Appendix E page 337). A more comprehensive list can be found on The 2-Day Diet website, which will help you calculate how much you are eating. Note that you will not be able to manage 24 g of fibre on the two restricted days, and typically will manage around 14 g. If you are not used to fibre in your diet it is best to increase your fibre intake gradually over two or three weeks – eating more fibre will inevitably create more gas and consuming too much fibre too quickly can lead to bloating, discomfort and flatulence. Make sure you drink more fluids when you increase your fibre intake – at least eight glasses of water or other low-calorie drinks daily.

Dairy foods

Like eggs, dairy foods have had a bad press in recent years. The claims that dairy foods can cause breast cancer have led many women to stop eating them, although despite extensive research, there is no evidence of a causal link. And for dieters, low-fat dairy foods are a positive asset. Milk protein seems to be particularly filling and there's evidence that the calcium in dairy foods acts almost like a detergent, grabbing fat before it can be absorbed – it's only a small effect but it probably amounts to around 45 calories a day that you don't have to lose elsewhere in your diet. The calcium in dairy foods may also benefit blood pressure and is vital for bone health. We've ensured that The 2-Day Diet is high in protein, calcium, vitamin D and fruit and vegetables, which all help maintain healthy bones. This is important since there is an inevitable small reduction in bone density when you diet as you are lighter and your bones are carrying less weight. Don't forget that weight-bearing exercise is also an essential part of keeping bones strong (see page 123).

Aim to have at least 800 mg of calcium a day – that's the equivalent of 200 ml (⅓ pint) of milk, one yoghurt and half a tin of salmon, provided you eat the bones too. If you don't enjoy, or are intolerant to, dairy products, make sure that you are getting plenty of calcium elsewhere in your diet (see below).

Calcium Ready-Reckoner

Food	Calcium (mg)
Sardines (tinned), if you eat the bones (100 g/3½ oz)	500
Pilchards (tinned), if you eat the bones (100 g/3½ oz)	300
Salmon (tinned), if you eat the bones (100 g/3½ oz)	300
Low-fat cheese such as Edam or low-fat Cheddar (30 g/1 oz)	240
Soya, rice, hazelnuts, oat milks (calcium-fortified) (200 ml/7 fl oz)	240
Fruit juice with added calcium (200 ml/7 fl oz)	240
Semi-skimmed or skimmed milk (200 ml/7 fl oz)	235
Yoghurt (150 g/5 oz)	225
Fromage frais (150 g/5 oz)	165
Purple sprouting broccoli (raw) (80 g/2½ oz)	160
Spinach, spring greens or curly kale (steamed) (100 g/3½ oz)	150
Okra (raw) (80 g/2½ oz)	130
Cottage cheese (100 g/3½ oz)	125
Soya yoghurt (calcium-fortified) (110 g)	120

Food	Calcium (mg)
Prawns (raw or boiled) (100 g/3½ oz)	110
Tofu (100 g/3½ oz)*	100*
Baked beans (½ tin) (210 g/7½ oz)	100
Red kidney beans (½ drained tin/120 g/4 oz)	85
Dried figs (30 g/1 oz)	80
Wholemeal bread (2 medium slices) (80 g/2½ oz)	75
Orange (160 g/5½ oz)	75
Almonds (30 g/1 oz)	70
Watercress (30 g/1 oz)	50
Broccoli (raw) (80 g/2½ oz)	45
Sweet potato (raw or cooked) (180 g/6 oz)	45
Cabbage (raw or cooked) (80 g/2½ oz)	40
Peas (fresh or frozen) (80 g/2½ oz)	30
Green beans and French beans (raw or cooked) (80 g/2½ oz)	30
Egg	30
Rhubarb (stewed) 3 tablespoons (80 g/2½ oz)	30
Apricots or currants (dried) (30 g/1 oz)	30
Red lentils (dried) (45 g/1½ oz)	25

* The amount of calcium in tofu is widely variable between brands. Make sure you choose tofu that has been set with calcium and contains calcium in the ingredients.

How to eat less salt

Too much salt can have a damaging effect on your health – it can raise your blood pressure and put you at higher risk of heart disease and stroke, and encourage loss of calcium from the bones, increasing the risk of osteoporosis. Current guidelines recommend no more than 6 g per day (about a teaspoon) – yet the average person in the UK consumes 8 g per day[8]. Many experts believe that we would be healthier if we cut down to just 3 g per day. About three-quarters of salt is hidden in the food we buy, especially processed foods such as ready meals, tinned soups, sausages, pizzas and takeaways. When buying food check the label for the salt content per 100 g – low salt is less than 0.3 g salt or 0.1 g sodium, medium is 0.3–1.5 g or 0.1–0.6 g sodium, high is over 1.5 g salt or 0.6 g sodium.

How to cut down your salt intake

- Limit your intake of ready meals and ready-made sauces.
- Cut down on salty snacks such as crisps and salted nuts.
- Avoid adding extra salt while cooking or at the table. Flavour with black pepper, fresh or dried herbs, or lemon juice instead.
- Choose reduced-salt versions of baked beans and soups.
- Choose tinned vegetables and pulses in water.
- Limit your intake of salty fish such as kippers and smoked salmon and salty meat products such as bacon and ham.

A word on food labelling

It's always good to know what is in the food you buy, especially when you're following a diet. You don't need to count calories on The 2-Day Diet, but you may want to check food labels. Currently two main types of food labelling are in common use.

Traffic light labelling

This shows you at a glance whether the fat, saturated fat, salt and sugar content of the food is low (green), medium (amber) or high (red). If you buy a food with all green lights you know immediately that it's a healthier choice.

Guideline Daily Amounts (GDAs)

GDAs indicate the approximate amount of nutrients or calories that an average person requires for a healthy diet. GDA labelling shows the contribution, expressed as a percentage, that the particular nutrients and calories in that food make to the overall GDA. So, for example, a yoghurt may be labelled with how much fat, sugar, salt, saturated fat and calories it contains and what percentage this contributes to the guideline daily amount for these nutrients.

Although the Food Standards Agency (FSA) encourages food manufacturers to use the traffic light system, many prefer GDAs, which are much more difficult to interpret. An updated voluntary traffic light system is being launched in 2013 in the hope that more manufacturers will sign up to it. The new labelling on the front of each food packet will combine the two existing systems so that you can see whether foods are high, medium or low in certain nutrients as traffic lights, as well as showing the percentage they contribute to the GDA.

How useful are they for the dieter?

Since both systems are based on an 'average' adult it is important to remember that these assessments may not be correct for you. Your recommended intakes may be lower, especially if you are following The 2-Day Diet and want to lose weight. Neither system includes all beneficial nutrients; for example they won't help you to choose a high-fibre food or one containing omega-3 fats.

Your questions answered

'What about transfats?'

Transfats are fats that naturally occur in small amounts in meat. Until recently the main dietary source of transfats was manufactured foods containing unsaturated fats that had been processed (hydrogenated) to become saturated. This was done to help solidify and preserve foods such as margarines, biscuits, cakes, crisps and crackers.

Transfats are bad for our health and have been linked to heart disease. Thankfully, as a result of pressure from consumers and the government, many manufacturers have removed transfats from foods in the UK. They are still present in a small number of foods, though, so check the ingredients and avoid foods that have hydrogenated or partially hydrogenated vegetable fat listed in the ingredients.

'Should I be sticking to low GI foods?'

Some diets focus on low Glycaemic Index (GI) foods as a way to lose weight and you will see GI ratings on some food labels. A food's GI score measures how quickly blood sugar rises when you eat that food and only applies to carbohydrates. Foods such as meat and cheese don't have a GI rating. The GI of foods is ranked from 0 to 100 (with sugar at 100).

High GI foods are broken down rapidly and they raise the blood sugar quickly, while low GI foods are digested slowly and gradually release sugar into the bloodstream. However, to make matters more complicated, the impact of the food on blood sugar depends not just on its GI, but also the amount of carbohydrate it contains (known as the Glycaemic Load). Some foods with a high GI such as watermelon (GI 72) contain very little carbohydrate, so will have a minimal effect on blood sugar. On top of that the GI of carbohydrate foods only tells you what happens when the food is eaten in isolation and this rarely happens – the GI is lowered, for example, when carbohydrate foods are eaten in combination with protein and fat. In addition, not all low GI foods are healthy – chocolate and ice cream, for example, have a low GI! It can be extremely confusing, so our recommendation is to forget GI – just aim to have a high-fibre diet and unrefined foods.

'Are sweeteners safe?'

There are two main types of sweetener. Intense sweeteners such as aspartame and sucralose are far sweeter than sugar and tend to be used in soft drinks. There is some concern that they may increase appetite and upset the beneficial balance of gut bacteria, although this is still unclear. Bulk sweeteners such as xylitol and sorbitol contain half the calories of sugar and are used in confectionery to add volume and texture as well as sweetness. High doses of these (more than 30 g/1 oz per day) can cause symptoms of nausea, diarrhoea and may also upset the balance of gut bacteria, although more research is needed. Any sweetener used in food in the EU has to undergo rigorous safety testing and have an agreed acceptable daily intake level (ADI), which incorporates a big safety margin.

Although the current guideline for aspartame is to consume less than 40 mg daily – equivalent to about 12 cans of a diet drink – the findings of two recent studies raise concerns that aspartame may be linked with certain blood cancers, which has sounded a note of caution with respect to their use. The links were seen both in animal studies, where consumption was equivalent to six cans of diet drink per day, and in a popu-lation study where intakes of more than 3 litres (6 pints) of diet drinks per week were linked to higher rates of blood cancers in men but not women[9]. Although these are preliminary find- ings, it makes sense to limit your intake of diet drinks to no more than 3 litres (6 pints), i.e. nine cans of diet drinks per week (see page 56). Don't be tempted to replace 'diet drinks' with sugary drinks, which are bad for both your health and your weight. In the study above sugary drinks were as strongly linked to blood cancer as diet drinks.

Am I allowed any alcohol?

You can have an occasional alcoholic drink, but try not to drink more than ten units a week, and none on the two restricted days of The 2-Day Diet (see table overleaf to see how many units of alcohol are in a typical drink). Alcohol deliv- ers double trouble for the dieter. It's packed with calories – a 250 ml (8½ fl oz) glass of wine contains 260 calories and a standard 'alcopop' 200 calories – and it makes you less inhibited, so you are more likely to give in to the temptation to eat! We know that alcohol consumed before or with meals makes you eat more. Even an aperitif can increase intake by 30 per cent[10]. While drinking a little may help protect against heart disease, alcohol can increase the risk of several different cancers including breast, bowel, liver, mouth and oesophageal cancer. The best choice, with fewest calories, is a spirit and diet-mixer (for example gin and slimline tonic, whisky and diet cola or vodka and diet lemonade). Decide on the maximum you are going to drink before you go out for the evening. Start with a low-cal soft drink or water and avoid salty snacks, which make you thirsty (and are usually full of calories). Try to drink more low-cal soft drinks or fizzy water than alcohol.

Alcohol	Units	Calories
Glass of wine 13% (250 ml/8½ fl oz)	3.3	240
Cider (568 ml/1 pint bottle)	2.3	210
Pint of beer/lager 4% (568 ml/1 pint)	2.3	170
Glass of wine 13% (175 ml/6 fl oz)	2.3	170
Champagne (125 ml/4 fl oz)	1.5	100
Alcopop 5% (275 ml/9 fl oz bottle)	1.4	200
Port (50 ml/1¾ fl oz)	1	79
Sherry (50 ml/1¾ fl oz)	1	58
Gin and slimline tonic (25 ml/1 fl oz gin*)	1	50

* A standard pub measure not home-poured.

'Should I cut out caffeine?'

Many people assume that decaffeinated tea or coffee is 'healthier' and that caffeine may raise blood pressure and increase the risk of heart disease. In fact there's no evidence that tea and coffee, caffeinated or otherwise, are bad for your health. Both can be a satisfying drink that can fend off the urge for a snack. Experts agree that for most people there is no clear association between caffeine consumption and the risk of high blood pressure or heart disease[11], although for people with high blood pressure, caffeine might cause a further slight, temporary increase. Both tea and coffee are packed with disease-fighting antioxidants, which can lower your risk of heart disease and certain cancers. And as long as you are getting enough calcium, caffeine isn't bad for bones: in fact the polyphenols in tea and coffee may actually be protective.

You might prefer to drink decaff because caffeinated drinks stop some people sleeping. Decaffeinated versions still contain beneficial antioxidants and there are no obvious concerns with the chemicals used in the decaffeination process.

It does, however, make sense to limit your intake of tea, coffee and other caffeinated drinks to no more than half of your total drinks during the day because they are diuretics, so they make you produce more urine and lose water. A recent review concluded that it is safe to consume 400 mg of caffeine per day with no adverse effects. Pregnant women should consume no more than 200 mg caffeine per day (see box below) while children should consume no more than 2.5 mg per kg body weight/day[12].

What is your caffeine intake?

- 1 mug of brewed coffee (125 mg)
- 1 mug of instant coffee (100 mg)
- 1 mug of tea (65 mg)
- 1 can of diet cola drink (40 mg)
- 30 g (1 oz) of 70% plain chocolate (24 mg)

'Is it safe to eat oily fish?'

Fish is good for you and is an important part of your 2-Day Diet – especially oily fish, which is one of our few dietary sources of vitamin D. However, current advice from the NHS and FSA is to limit certain types of fish because they contain low levels of environmental pollutants such as dioxins and PCBs or mercury, which can be harmful if they build up in the body. Try not to eat more than four servings of oily fish and certain white fish and seafood (sea bream, sea bass, turbot, halibut, rock salmon and brown crab) per week. Children, or anyone who is, or is planning to become, pregnant should restrict themselves to two servings per week. Children and women who are pregnant or planning to become pregnant should also avoid swordfish, shark and marlin completely and everyone else should restrict themselves to one serving of these fish a week as they can contain mercury. You can safely eat unlimited amounts of fish such as cod, haddock, plaice, pollock, coley, dover sole, dab, flounder, red mullet, gurnard and white crab meat.

'Can I still have treats?'

We found that our 2-Day Dieters fell into two groups – those who were keen to include treats as part of the Diet because it made it feel less restrictive and those who felt that it was important to cut out chocolate and other sweet snacks. Only you will know what works for you, but remember that restricting a food can lead to cravings and wanting to binge on it. If you want to include some treats as part of your Diet, we recommend limiting them to three servings a week (see the table opposite). Note that some foods that are often thought of as healthy, such as flapjacks, are very high in calories – so a 'treat' is only two 'mini bites' (3 cm/1 in square).

If you don't think you can live without chocolate, don't worry. Although you can't have chocolate on your two restricted days of The 2-Day Diet, it's fine to have a bit of chocolate, or another 'treat' food during the five unrestricted days. Chocolate is high in calories, sugar and saturated fat, so don't overdo it (see opposite for recommended amounts) and choose a dark chocolate that's high in cocoa solids (70–85 per cent) that may help reduce blood pressure and improve blood sugar control. In fact a recent study allocated women to eat either 20 g (⅔ oz) of 80 per cent dark chocolate a day or 20 g (⅔ oz) of standard milk chocolate every day for four weeks. The good news was that women eating the 80 per cent chocolate saw a reduction in their blood pressure and insulin levels; however, the milk chocolate group saw quite the opposite effect and these women had a 20 per cent reduction in the efficiency of their insulin[13].

Treat	Servings
Low-fat crisps	1 small packet (25–30 g/¾–1 oz)
Plain or chocolate biscuits (e.g. digestive)	2
Chocolate (ideally dark > 70% cocoa)	5 small squares or 30 g (1 oz)
Ice cream	2 scoops (100 g/3½ oz) standard or 1 scoop (50 g/1¾ oz) luxury
Malt loaf	1 slice
Hot cross bun	1 bun
Fruity teacake	1 teacake
Fairy cakes	2 small cakes with thin or no icing
Flapjack	2 'mini bites' (3 cm/1 in square)
Jaffa cakes or small chocolate chip	3 cookies
Individual chocolate or truffle	3

Snack ideas for the five unrestricted days of the week

- Oatcakes, rye crispbreads or wholemeal crackers with low-fat hummus, low-fat cream cheese or cottage cheese.
- Fruit.

- Vegetable crudités, such as celery, cucumber, green peppers, mange tout, spring onions and cherry tomatoes, with salsa, low-fat hummus, tuna pâte, tsatsiki or guacamole. (see pages 194–196)
- Plain, diet or fruit yoghurt.
- Malt loaf, with or without margarine or low-fat spread.
- Small handful of unsalted nuts (for example, walnuts, pistachio nuts or Brazil nuts) or dried fruit (for example, apricots, figs, sultanas or mango).
- A glass of vegetable juice (carrot, tomato, or mixture).
- Plain popcorn (popped in vegetable oil with no sugar or salt added).
- Bowl of soup (see pages 250–256).
- Smoothie made with skimmed or semi-skimmed milk, yoghurt and one piece of fruit.
- Dried pea snacks.
- Sugar-free jelly.
- Ice lolly made from frozen, diluted, sugar-free squash.

Summary

▶ The five unrestricted days of The 2-Day Diet are based on a healthy Mediterranean diet with lots of vegetables, wholegrains, beans, fish, pulses, fruit, nuts and healthy oils and can include small amounts of lean, red meat.

▶ Eating foods that are high in soluble and insoluble fibre will help keep you full and keep your blood sugar stable and your bowels healthy.

▶ Make sure you still have plenty of healthy protein foods on the five unrestricted days of The 2-Day Diet as this will help to fill you up and stop you overeating. This will maximise your weight loss with The 2-Day Diet.

▶ Low-fat dairy foods help fill you up and keep your bones strong.

▶ It's important to stay well-hydrated and drink at least eight glasses of fluid a day.

▶ You are allowed occasional treats such as alcohol and chocolate, but limit them to two or three times a week.

5

making The 2-Day Diet work

You've made the decision to start The 2-Day Diet and you're on your way. The focus of this chapter is to lay the groundwork that will make sure you have the best chance of success, help you to deal with any problems that might arise and to answer your diet questions.

Eight steps to successful weight loss

Step one: plan ahead

Prepare a shopping list before you set out to do your weekly shop – and stick to it. If you have the right foods at home, you're more likely to persevere with The 2-Day Diet, but if your cupboards are stuffed with temptations like biscuits, crisps and chocolate you will be making your life much harder. 'Out of sight' really is 'out of mind' and craving-inducing comfort foods are much easier to avoid if they aren't around to tempt you. One study found that simply moving dishes of sweets from people's desks to the other side of the room meant that they ate less of them[1]. If you keep snacks in the cupboard 'for the kids' and often end up tucking into them yourself, ask yourself whether it's time to get these snacks out of the house and improve the children's diets too. If not (if you can't face the mutiny!), store them in a special container marked 'Kids only!'

Try the following tips:

▶ Never go food-shopping on an empty stomach: it is too tempting to buy (and then eat) things that you'll regret later.

▶ Pack a healthy home-made lunch to take to work and keep healthy snacks (if you're likely to need them) in your office drawer, handbag or car to help you avoid the temptation of eating things that you shouldn't. For ideas see the meal plans in chapter 8 (see pages 170–179).

▶ Don't be afraid to let people know that you're trying to lose weight and would prefer not to have chocolate, sweets or cakes as gifts, or for them to persuade you to indulge if you meet them for a coffee.

▶ Ask your friends and family to actively support your weight-loss efforts (see page 36). Talk it up and let the important people in your life know how you're doing and feeling. If you're struggling and need some encouragement, don't beat around the bush – just ask for it.

▶ Visit www.thetwodaydiet.co.uk for further information, support and tips or find us on Facebook to connect with other 2-Day Dieters and to share your experiences.

'I've always had a thing for pastry, chocolate and cakes and the lack of them is the only negative about the diet. But I'm adapting well now that I understand the effects they are having on my body and my health.' Susie, 35

Step two: watch your liquid calories

Drinks can work for or against you. Having a glass of water or another non-calorie drink when you are eating a meal has been shown to reduce the amount you eat[2], but some drinks are loaded with calories. A 330 ml (11 fl oz) can of regular cola contains 145 calories – whereas the diet version only contains one calorie. What's more, these fluid calories bypass normal appetite controls, making it all too easy to consume too many. If you need fizzy drinks in your life, include an occasional diet drink in your eating plan. Despite some concerns there's no convincing evidence that these can increase osteoporosis risk by leaching calcium from the bones as long as you are getting enough calcium in your diet.

The same applies to other drinks – a couple of lattes can really bump up your calorie count, even if you go for the skinny version. A large full-fat milk latte comes in at a whopping 223 calories, while the skimmed-milk version still contains 131 calories. By contrast an Americano with semi-skimmed milk contains only 20 calories, so drink coffee or tea with a splash of milk or herbal teas instead.

Step three: beware of portion distortion

Most of us have noticed that serving sizes have grown massively over the last few decades and are getting larger as food companies and outlets want to sell us more food and we have become used to these larger portions. Twenty years ago a medium slice of bread weighed 30 g (1 oz) and contained 65 calories; today it weighs 45 g (1½ oz) and contains 90 calories. Similarly, hot cross buns have grown in size from 50 g (1¾ oz) to 75 g (2½ oz) and from 155 to 220 calories.

Many high-calorie snack foods are two, or even three, times as big as they were 30 years ago – and that means twice or three times the calories. Researchers have shown that when we are presented with servings that are bigger than we need, most of us will eat more without even thinking about it[3]. The good news is that, conversely, if we're given smaller servings and fewer calories we will eat less without feeling deprived[4]. That's why, as well as telling you the types of food to eat, The 2-Day Diet provides clear guidelines on the amounts to eat for dieting success. This should not be an issue on the two restricted days of The 2-Day Diet, when the high-protein foods mean that you tend to self-limit what you eat. We certainly don't expect you to weigh all your foods – we provide simple guidelines for gauging portion sizes alongside weights of food servings on both the two restricted days and the five unrestricted days of The 2-Day Diet. Many of our 2-Day Dieters did find it helpful to weigh foods such as breakfast cereals, pasta and rice, which are easy to pour out and overdo, until they got used to the recommended serving sizes.

'Being able to vary the restricted days of The 2-Day Diet means I can fit them around social occasions and holidays, so I don't feel as though I'm missing out.' Jane, 49

Step four: sit at a table to eat

Eating on the run, or while you are watching TV, sitting at your desk or at your computer, or even listening to the radio, means that you are focusing on something else and you will tend to consume more calories – simply because you don't notice what or how much you are eating[5]. In one study people eating crisps while watching TV ate around 40 per cent more than on another occasion when they didn't watch any TV[6].

The best way to avoid uncontrolled munching is to sit down at a table, eat slowly and savour each mouthful – without doing something else, such as watching TV, at the same time. It takes about 15 minutes for your brain to let your stomach know that you have eaten enough, so make yourself wait at least 15 minutes after finishing a meal to decide whether you are still hungry and whether you really need seconds or dessert.

> *'The 2-Day Diet suited me, as it taught me to eat the correct food types and experiment with different foods. I've been losing the inches. Trousers that were tight are now comfortable and I don't get that bloated feeling.'*
> Ruth, 53

Step five: avoid 'diet' foods

The supermarkets are full of them – the low-fat, low-sugar 'diet' foods that promise an easy way to eat fewer calories and lose weight. We don't recommend basing your diet on these highly processed diet foods, but to stick to the whole and unprocessed foods we recommend on the restricted and unrestricted days of The 2-Day Diet. Of course it can be helpful knowing the calorie content of foods. Don't forget that calories will be listed per 100 g or per 100 ml or per product, so you will need to multiply this up (or down) to work out you how many calories are in each serving.

Don't mistake 'low fat' for 'low calorie'. A lot of foods labelled 'light', 'lite' or 'lower fat' can still contain quite large amounts of fat and, therefore, calories. Manufacturers often replace the fat in low-fat foods with sugar to improve the flavour, so these foods can provide just as many calories and often contain fructose (see page 73). The only 'diet' foods that may be useful are low-fat foods and those that use artificial sweeteners with no added sugar, such as diet drinks. Remember to stay within the limit of no more than 3 litres (6 pints, i.e. nine cans) of diet drink per week.

Step six: manage your expectations

Stick to the rules of The 2-Day Diet, follow the exercise guidelines (see chapter 6) and we promise that you will achieve successful – and rapid – weight loss. That said, it won't happen overnight and you might experience a few setbacks. You will be burning fat on the two restricted days of The 2-Day Diet but you will notice a drop in your weight during and immediately afterwards as you also lose water – typically between 1–2 lb (0.5 kg–1 kg) over the two days. Fat-burning is a complex process and most people won't lose any more than 4½ lb (2 kg) of fat per week. Any weight loss beyond this will just be loss of water.

If you think back to how long it has taken you to put on your excess weight, you have to be realistic and realise that it will take a while to get rid of it too. A pound (0.5 kg) of body fat contains around 4,500 calories so, in theory, to lose a pound of fat in a week you should burn off or consume 4,500 fewer calories – around 640 fewer calories per day. Unfor- tunately it's not that simple, because when you diet, your metabolic rate falls and your body adapts to a lower calorie intake. Research that monitored calorie intake and expendi- ture (from resting metabolic rate and activity) and fat loss found that to lose one pound of fat per week, on average, you actually need to eat 850 calories less than you need each day[7]. This is a lot of calories and by far the best way to achieve it is through a combination of diet and exercise. If you do 30 minutes of exercise five times a week you only need to eat 700 fewer calories per day to lose the weight. If you exercise for an hour five times a week you would only have to eat 550 fewer calories. You might feel a bit disappointed by the fact that exercise burns so few calories, but remember that exercise improves overall health and reduces risks of many diseases (see page 119). What's more we consistently find that exercise appears to help Dieters adhere better to their weight-loss diet.

'I am 30 years old and have lost just over 7 lb (3 kg) in three weeks. I noticed results within about a week. Every winter I always tend to grow my 'winter coat' (i.e. put on a few pounds from eating comfort food!). This diet has really helped me to drop the weight, which I have been unable to shift through exercise and other diets.' Sally, 30

Step seven: monitor your progress

Monitoring is a vital part of any weight-loss plan. We know that Dieters who monitor themselves do better. The way you feel in your clothes will give you clues about what's happening to your weight, but you should still weigh yourself and measure your waist and hips once a week and make a note of the results. You can use these measurements to reassess your percentage body fat and weight of body fat – ideally every two weeks – using the ready reckoner in Appendix A (pages 314–315).

How to monitor yourself

- Weight can fluctuate from day to day (up or down by 2–4½ lb/1–2 kg), so it is not a good idea to weigh yourself every day as this could give you a skewed picture of your overall progress.
- Weight can change throughout the day, so always weigh and measure yourself at the same time of day (ideally first thing in the morning as we are usually heavier at the end of the day) and before eating a meal.
- Use the same set of reliable scales. Don't stand bathroom scales on an uneven or soft surface such as a carpet – most bathroom scales work best when placed on a hard, level floor.
- Remove your clothes and shoes before weighing yourself or wear light layers only.
- Measure your waist and hips without clothes on as some clothes can be constricting and give unreliable, sometimes misleading, measurements.
- For women, weight and waist measurements are often greater just before your period because of fluid retention – you may see gains of 4½ lb (2 kg) and even up to 11 lb (5 kg), depending on how much you weigh.
- Because you will lose water on the two restricted days of The 2-Day Diet we suggest that you weigh yourself immediately before and not after your restricted days each week. If you step on the scales immediately after the two days you will be lighter as you will have lost fluid as well as some fat.

*'I eat out a lot and in the past restaurants have always
been the scene of my diet-breaking crimes, but it's
definitely been possible to choose from a normal menu –
even on a restricted day. I've probably had to eat out on
at least one of my two restricted days each week since I
started the diet and I'm still seeing brilliant results. This
has to be the easiest diet to fit around your real life.'*
Alison, 26

Step eight: reward your success

Although your final reward – reaching your weight-loss goal
– is some way down the line, it's important to recognise and
reward yourself for even small successes on the way. Losing
weight takes focus and commitment and you deserve regular
pats on the back for your hard work. You should have already
set yourself short-term weight-loss and exercise goals. Setting
up a reward system adds an extra incentive, prevents you
getting bored and gives you something to work towards.

Rewards are a very personal thing and only you know
what would be a real treat for you – although treats should
obviously not involve food or alcohol! This could be your
opportunity to use the money you've saved on The 2-Day
Diet to treat yourself (see page 68). Buy yourself some new
clothes or that new pair of boots or shoes you've been long-
ing for; arrange to have a facial, manicure, pedicure or have a
new haircut; book a day off work and just take it easy; reserve
tickets for a film, play or show that you want to see. For men,
why not go for a spin on the karting track or get that new
gizmo for your toolbox that you've been hankering after?

CASE STUDY: Sarah

At over 14½ stone (92 kg) Sarah was desperate to lose weight. Her mum had been diagnosed with breast cancer in her forties and 10 years later the cancer had come back. A self- confessed chocoholic, Sarah, 39, knew that being overweight increased her risk of breast cancer. She tried slimming clubs and many different diets at home, but although she lost some weight, it always piled back on. By the time Sarah started The 2-Day Diet she had almost given up hope. 'I knew it would be a challenge, but I developed a routine, making the same two days each week my diet days and eating the same foods each week. I made the diet days my busiest work days so that I didn't miss eating. What surprised me was that I didn't want to overeat on my non-diet days – perhaps because I had become more aware of what I was eating. I lost a stone (6.4 kg) in the first month and over a six-month period lost 4 stone (25 kg). It is the easiest diet I have ever done.'

Your questions answered

'Is it important to eat at particular times of the day?'

When we eat is dictated by all sorts of things – family habits, social pressure and convenience – as well as actually feeling hungry. There is no conclusive evidence that eating earlier in the day, avoiding eating after a certain time in the evening or having smaller, more frequent, meals rather than large meals will have any impact on your metabolic rate and your body's ability to burn or store fat[8]. However, what is important is your individual response to the timing and the frequency of eating that may make you prone to overeating in certain situations. If you know that evenings are a time when you get the munchies, or that you find it hard not to eat a large dinner even if you aren't hungry, then it's important to become aware of this and to take precautions for times when you might overeat. Evenings are danger times for many people and it often helps to stay busy, for example you could sort out the newspapers, do the ironing or something practical with your hands (such as knitting) while watching TV. If tea and biscuits in front of the TV is your 'reward' after a hard day's work, but you can't stop at just one biscuit, find another way to reward yourself – with a long aromatic bath or an evening out. It also helps to brush your teeth after the last time you eat during the day – to signal to your body that eating is over for the day.

'Isn't eating after 5pm more fattening?'

Lots of people believe this, but science shows quite clearly that it's the total number of calories you consume over the 24 hours that determines whether you gain or lose weight. Food eaten in the evening is no more likely to be stored as fat than food eaten earlier in the day. A number of studies have found that food eaten late at night is processed in exactly the same way as the same food eaten as several small meals throughout the day[9].

'I've heard that lack of sleep can make you fat. Does it?'

We all have an internal body clock, which is controlled by our brain and which helps co-ordinate the hormones that control our appetite and the metabolism of food. Our body clocks are designed to function around our normal pattern of waking and sleeping, which, in turn, is fundamentally controlled by the cycle of daylight and darkness. If our lifestyle is at odds with this body clock it can affect our metabolism and weight control. Although this is a new area of research, there is emerging evidence that if you are someone who has less sleep and prefers to be up at night and eat most of your food at night, or someone who has to do this because of shift work, you could be a greater risk of gaining weight, due to increased appetite and possibly reductions in your metabolic rate and fat-burning.

Research consistently shows that having only five to six hours' sleep increases the appetite and daily calorie intake by 200 calories[10]. In a recent study conducted in a hotel-type setting in Boston, volunteers spent three weeks in conditions where they were allowed only five and a half hours' sleep per night. Their body clocks were disrupted through being denied daylight and being put onto a 28-hour cycle. After just three weeks their resting metabolic rate fell by 8 per cent – a drop that would translate into weight gain of around 13 lb (5.8 kg) over a year[11].

If you are a shift worker

Working shifts and dieting to lose weight takes more planning and self-discipline than if you work normal hours because some disruption to your body clock is inevitable. But it can be done – the recent brilliantly titled Australian POWER (Preventing Obesity Without Eating like a Rabbit!) study asked a group of male shift workers in an aluminium plant to followed a healthy calorie-controlled diet and included exercise using the tips below. It worked! After 14 weeks the men had lost, on average, nearly 9 lb (4 kg) and 4 cm (1½ in) from their waists[12].

Tips for shift workers

- If you work nights, eat a light meal during the night and a small breakfast when you finish work.
- Plan ahead to help you eat as healthily as possible, especially in situations where the food on offer tends to be high-calorie, greasy junk food. Take fruit and vegetables with you to snack on during your shift and limit your intake of fizzy and caffein-ated drinks. Drink water throughout your shift.
- Shift workers often struggle to get good-quality sleep. Make sure your bedroom is quiet, dark and not too warm. Close the curtains or blinds, wear earplugs and an eye mask if neces-sary. Make sure that your family and friends know that this is your 'night' and that you shouldn't be interrupted. Create a sleep schedule for yourself and stick to it, sleeping at the same time during the working week and at the weekends.
- Incorporate exercise into your breaks at work. Walk for 10 minutes and do some simple stretches.
- Fit cardiovascular and resistance exercises (see pages 123–124) into the time after you rest or wake up.
- Join a 24-hour gym if you want to work out during irregular hours. Run, walk, cycle, dance or do any activity that gets your heart rate up and burns calories.
- Talk to other shift workers and share tips on how to stay healthy while working shifts. Create or join a support group with your peers.

'Do I have to eat breakfast?'

We've all been told that a good breakfast is essential for physical and mental performance because your body hasn't been fed all night and it needs food to refuel. And it's often quoted as a vital meal for dieters as it will kick-start your metabolism and help to control overeating later in the day. While it's important that children have their breakfast, our advice is, don't force yourself to eat breakfast if you don't want it. Some of us are 'morning' people, who feel hungry and need breakfast to get going, but if you can't face breakfast first thing and so tend not to eat it, follow your appetite and wait until you are hungry. When researchers from Roehampton University asked men who didn't normally eat breakfast to include it, they didn't eat less for the rest of the day – in fact they ate 300 calories more than normal. But when people who always ate breakfast were asked to skip it, they overate later in the day[13]. The take-home message is that we are probably all wired differently, so do what feels right for you. If you are a breakfast-eater, it doesn't have to be toast and cereal – a high-protein break-fast, such as eggs, will help you feel fuller for longer. When researchers compared an egg-based, 400-calorie breakfast with a 400-calorie carbohydrate-based breakfast (bagels in this case), the egg-eaters consumed 400 fewer calories during the day than the bagel-eaters[14].

'I have tried to lose weight so many times before that I don't know whether it's worth trying again. Has dieting messed up my metabolism?'

We have found The 2-Day Diet to be successful, not just for first-time dieters but for people who have tried, time after time, to lose weight. Some of our Dieters had more than 10 previous attempts at dieting. Researchers at the Fred Hutchinson Cancer Research Centre in Seattle found that 'yo-yo' dieters who had tried and failed to lose weight three or more times previously were just as able to lose weight and see

reductions in insulin and inflammation in the body (the anti-
cipated beneficial effect of weight loss) as dieters who hadn't
ever been on a diet[15].

A word about snacking

To snack or not to snack? It's a topic of endless debate. Some
people argue that snacking helps to control your appetite
because it stops you getting really hungry and then overeating at
mealtimes. Others say that snacking just encourages you to keep
focusing on food and makes you eat more. We often see dieters
who have previously tried to eat something religiously every hour
or so, believing it will boost their metabolism, although this is not
the case.

There is no evidence that snacking between meals is better for
controlling hunger or reducing levels of 'appetite' hormones. And
there is no difference in your metabolic rate whether you eat two
large meals, or six or seven smaller ones a day if you consume
the same amount overall. It's possible that you may burn less
body fat after a large meal, but the impact of this will be extremely
small[16].

At the end of the day how many meals you eat really depends
on you and the bottom line is not when you eat, but how much
you eat in total within the 24-hour day. You probably know the
pattern of eating that suits you best and helps control your appetite. If not, experiment with it and see whether it works better for
you to stick with two or three large meals, or to have five or six
smaller ones.

It might be worth remembering that as long as you don't over- eat,
there may actually be health benefits in leaving longer periods
between eating. We know that beneficial changes occur when our

cells are not constantly fed with calories (see page 18). So leaving longer gaps between meals, when your cells aren't being 'fed', may have a beneficial effect. For most of us this happens every night as we have 12 hours without food between our last meal of the day and breakfast – although it may not happen if you are up snacking in front of the TV until 2am and eat a big breakfast at 7am when you get up.

SWAP IT! See how many calories you could save!	
✘	✔
Can of cola and chocolate muffin (465 calories)	Diet cola and apple (45 calories)
Bar of milk chocolate (280 calories)	Diet yoghurt (100 calories)
Packet of crisps (160 calories)	Vegetable sticks and low-calorie dip (25 calories)

'Help – I've broken my diet!'

Even the most dedicated dieter slips up from time to time – and the slip-up is usually eating 'forbidden' foods. This is one reason why we have made sure there are treats on The 2-Day Diet! If you do slip up, don't beat yourself up about it or feel like a failure – and certainly don't give up. Dieting lapses happen to everyone and the best thing you can do is to get back on track as soon as you can. For our 2-Day Dieters, holidays were the biggest danger times. Some also struggled when they were stressed, short of time, in the run-up to their period or when they found themselves in certain social situations. Even though you are unrestricted for five days out of seven each week, there may be times when it is helpful to prescribe yourself a diet 'break', which can be a good way to deal with high-risk periods or to combat diet boredom. One recent study looked at the impact of a planned two-week diet 'holiday' on people's long-term success. The result? After the break the dieters managed to successfully return to their diets and it did not hamper their long-term success[17]. If you know that you have an event or a special occasion coming up, think ahead and plan to deviate from the Diet temporarily and then get back on track afterwards – rather than convincing yourself that you will not be tempted on the day and then being disappointed with yourself when you do.

Don't forget, if you do lapse, try to learn from the experience to enable you to avoid doing the same thing the next time – ask yourself: 'What was the situation?', 'How did I respond?', 'How did I feel afterwards?' and 'What could I do differently next time?'

'Why is my weight loss slowing down?'

Weight loss becomes harder when you have been dieting for a while, usually after about six months have gone by. Part of this may be due to the inevitable 10–15 per cent reduction in metabolic rate that happens as your body adapts to weight loss and eating less (even when you exercise). But weight loss often slows down because you may not be sticking as carefully to the Diet or exercising as much as when you first started.

If you feel you are not losing the predicted 1–2 lb (0.5 kg –1 kg) per week, check the following:

▶ Are you following the correct diet plan for someone of your sex, weight, and age (see Appendix D, pages 328–336)?

▶ Are you overeating on the two restricted days of The 2-Day Diet?

▶ Are you overeating on the five unrestricted days of The 2-Day Diet or drinking too much alcohol?

▶ Are you taking the recommended amount of exercise (see chapter 6)?

▶ Are you taking every opportunity to be physically active in your daily routine? For example taking the stairs or aiming to walk rather than drive, where possible?

▶ Keep a tally of your food servings and log your activity diary for four days to check how much you are eating and how active you really are. Remember to include both weekdays and weekends.

'How do I beat my food cravings?'

Most of us have foods that we crave occasionally. Unfortunately when you are trying to diet, these cravings can become worse. Although some cravings are driven by hunger, many are triggered by internal cues – if you feel bored or anxious you might be in the habit of eating chocolate to make your- self feel better. You may also respond to external cues such as seeing chocolate by the till when you are buying your healthy salad lunch, seeing other people eat or certain social situations. Interestingly many of our 2-Day Dieters stopped craving chocolate and sweet treats, but sometimes craved bread, cereals and other carbohydrates on their two restricted days, which of course they were then able to eat on their five unrestricted days.

Try to identify your particular triggers. When are you most likely to feel those cravings and what are the common factors? Is it about the way you feel, what is happening around you or a combination of the two? The good news is that you can reprogramme your brain to overcome these urges. You may just have a craving to eat something – in which case try having a hot drink, a diet drink or perhaps some sugar-free mints or sugar-free chewing gum.

There are two approaches that can be helpful:

▶ **Distraction**. A food craving is like a wave that gets bigger and bigger, but then subsides. So while a craving can feel overwhelming – and irresistible – as it builds up, you need to remind yourself that it will pass. Try to ride it out by distracting yourself. You may find that the craving will go if you can distract yourself for 15 to 20 minutes by focusing on something else. Get busy with housework, phone a friend, go for a walk, have a shower or clean your teeth.

▶ **Acceptance** (feel the craving and work through it). Let yourself experience the full force of the craving, be really conscious of it and try to notice what you are thinking and feeling, without giving in to it. This approach may be harder initially, but learning that you can manage to resist the urge to eat the food you crave can give you a real sense of achievement and make it easier next time, because you know that you are able to take control and make choices about what you eat[18].

How can I stop myself comfort-eating?'

Many of us overeat when we are stressed or depressed. Although eating can give you a quick fix, in the longer term comfort-eating doesn't provide much comfort, especially if you're trying to lose weight, and it often leaves you feeling more anxious and stressed. The key here is to recognise when you are stressed and find ways to manage it (see page 38).

'I always get the munchies before my period. What should I do?'

The week before the start of a period is a difficult time for many women. As well as feeling moody and anxious, it's common to experience cravings, especially for high-carbohydrate foods. It's thought that these cravings are due to your body trying to take in enough carbohydrate to balance levels of chemicals in the brain.

About half of our Dieters had difficulty managing pre-menstrual syndrome (PMS) cravings on the two restricted days of The 2-Day Diet – we suggest that you experiment and see how you feel. If it's too difficult to do your two restricted days when you are pre-menstrual, try to reschedule these days for when you're not suffering from PMS.

Try to deal with carbohydrate cravings on the five unrestricted eating days by eating wholegrain rather than refined carbohydrates (see page 74). Calcium, magnesium and vitamin B6 are all thought to help reduce PMS and suppress cravings[19], so eat plenty of foods rich in these nutrients (see www.thetwodaydiet.co.uk). Calcium is found in low-fat dairy foods, eggs, spinach, green vegetables and tinned sardines, pilchards and salmon (including the bones); some good dietary sources of magnesium include wholegrain cereals and vegetables; and good sources of B6 include lean meat, eggs, wholegrain cereals, soya beans, peanuts and milk.

The good news is that many women find that their PMS improves when they lose weight and take regular exercise.

'I am prone to suffering from seasonal affective disorder (SAD) in winter. How can I curb my cravings?'

Many of us get a touch of the 'winter blues', when we feel low and lethargic during the winter months, but around half a million people in the UK suffer more severely and have what is known as seasonal affective disorder (SAD). This is caused by the lack of daylight affecting the chemical balance of the brain and reducing levels of serotonin, a chemical that promotes relaxation and happiness. SAD is more common among women, particularly those aged between 20 and 50. Whether you have the winter blues or full-blown SAD you will probably notice a craving for starchy and sugary foods, which both help boost levels of serotonin in the brain. So what is the answer? Exercise is a great therapy as it helps to restore the chemical balance of the brain and helps you to feel good about yourself. Walking outside for an hour a day has also been shown to help SAD sufferers.

We often find that people do better at losing weight in the summer, perhaps because low-calorie foods are more desirable and it's less tempting to have stodgy 'comfort' foods when the weather is warm and it's easier to get out and exercise. In the summer our Dieters lost, on average 15 lb (6.8 kg), whereas in the winter it was only 11½ lb (5.3 kg). This doesn't mean that you should delay starting your diet (and exercise) until the summer. Just be aware that losing weight may be more of a challenge – and if you do delay, this may mean another winter when you gain weight so that you eventually have more to lose when you do start dieting.

Eating out and takeaways

There will inevitably be times during your 2-Day Diet when you have to eat away from home because of work or social occasions. So how do you keep your 2-Day Diet on track?

- Meals out are usually bigger and higher in calories than meals at home, and they often contain lots of hidden fat. However, more restaurants and takeaway outlets are now informing customers about the calorie content of their foods, to help make people more aware of the healthier choices. So do make use of this information if it is available. Try to avoid fixed-price menus as you may well end up eating more courses and calories than you need or want – just because it's included in the price. Also, 'all you can eat' restaurants are probably best avoided – the temptation to pile your plate high just because you can is possibly too great!

- Don't starve yourself all day before you go out – you could overeat when you eventually sit down to your meal.

- Share courses with your companions, so that you don't overeat.

- Perhaps order just two starters instead of a starter plus a main course.

- Eat slowly and savour every mouthful.

- Don't be afraid to ask for exactly what you want by requesting that the menu is adapted. Most restaurants will be happy to do this.

- Ask for high-calorie sauces or dressings to be served on the side so that you can decide how much of them you put on your food.

- Don't be afraid to ask how the food is cooked if it is not clear from reading the menu. Most waiters are only too happy to explain these details.

- Be careful about eating lots of nibbles before the meal such as bread soaked in olive oil, crisps, poppadoms or prawn crackers as they add lots of extra calories.

- Drink plenty of water and less wine. Ordinary tap water should be freely available and will save money on your drinks bill, as well as keeping your calories down.
- The following words and phrases mean that extra fat and calories have been added: à la crème, au gratin, battered, Béarnaise, béchamel, beurre blanc, breaded, butter, crispy, cheese sauce, cordon bleu, creamed, en croûte, escalloped, flaky, florentine, fried, hollandaise, meunière, Milanese, pan-fried, Parmigiani, rich, sauté, tempura.

Summary

▶ Plan ahead, monitor your weight loss and exercise, and control your serving sizes to give yourself the best chance of success.

▶ Find the pattern of eating that works for you, whether it's eating a few large meals or several smaller ones each day.

▶ Successful weight loss takes time. Don't be disheartened if the weight doesn't fall off as quickly as you had hoped or if it slows down. If you keep to The 2-Day Diet you will succeed.

▶ Make sure you get enough sleep and manage your stress levels, as neglecting either can put you off track.

▶ Reward yourself for every success and don't be disappointed if things occasionally go wrong – just get back on The 2-Day Diet.

'Cutting back on my bread and potatoes means that I don't feel so stodged up. My stomach has shrunk, therefore I don't feel so hungry.' Georgina, 53

6

how to be more active

Getting moving and staying active will speed up your weight loss, enhance the health benefits of The 2-Day Diet and boost your mood and energy levels. The good news is that if you've been a confirmed couch potato up until now, it's never too late to start moving, and being active really doesn't have to be hard. Our 2-Day Dieters showed us that even if you've never exercised before, you can make physical activity a regular part of your life. We will show you how to start slowly, build up gradually and stay motivated so that you hit your weight-loss and fitness goals.

Why you need to get moving

Left to their own devices people tend to move less, rather than more, when they start dieting. Research shows that activity levels can drop by around 40 per cent when people go on a diet and when you move less you need fewer calories, which makes it harder to lose weight[1]. Get moving and it will have the reverse effect, helping to increase your weight loss as well as boost your health and help you to look and feel better.

You'll lose more weight

When you lose weight your metabolic rate falls because your body needs fewer calories in order to function. Exercise helps to combat this and keep your weight loss on track by burning extra calories. Exercise alone won't shift much extra weight – it's the combination of diet and exercise that really makes the difference. Research studies have shown people who only exercise and don't diet lose only 3 lb (1.4 kg), those who only diet and don't exercise lose 16½ lb (7.5 kg), but the real winners are those diet and exercise – they shed 21 lb (9.5 kg)[2].

You'll maintain calorie-burning muscle

Everyone loses muscle as well as fat when they lose weight, but exercise can halve that muscle loss. So if you lose 19 lb (8.6 kg) you will lose 6 lb (2.7 kg) of that as muscle if you're not exercising. With exercise you'll only lose 3 lb (1.4 kg) of muscle. Hanging on to that extra muscle is important for fat-burning because muscle burns seven times more calories than fat. One of the major effects of ageing is to lose muscle and the average Western woman loses about ½ lb (0.3 kg) of muscle every year. Exercising while you diet will reduce the rate of the ageing process and save you six years of normal muscle loss.

'I was a bit worried that exercising on my restricted days would make me hungrier and struggle to keep to the diet. Actually, going swimming after work gives me a routine, keeps me on track and avoids the evening munchies.'

Pat, 54

Your body will love it!

Our bodies are designed to move – and when they don't they suffer. Bones and muscles become weaker and your heart and lungs become less efficient at pumping blood around your body. Becoming active can actually boost your immune system, helping to protect you against viral infections and colds. A single exercise session can lower your blood pressure, increase the effectiveness of your insulin (this is called 'insulin sensitivity') and lower the levels of harmful fats in your blood for 24 to 48 hours[3]. Being active for 150 minutes a week – that's just half an hour, five days a week – reduces your risk of type 2 diabetes, cuts heart disease and stroke risk by 30 per cent and cuts your risk of dying prematurely from any cause by 50 per cent[4]. The health benefits of taking up exercise are considered as important as giving up smoking. Moving a bit more – three to four hours a week – can cut your risk of breast and colon cancer by 30 per cent. On top of that, exercise will benefit your bones and joints, helping to protect you against osteoporosis and arthritis.

'I always find I can keep to my diet better when I am also being active. A brisk walk or run can really boost my mood and make me determined not to overeat.'

Rachel, 44

Your mood will improve

You won't just feel the physical benefits of exercise, it can help to energise you, help you sleep better, alleviate depression and stimulate the release of feel-good brain chemicals that help you feel happier and more relaxed. In fact, exercise combats many of the things that can make us overeat in the first place – stress, depression and low self-esteem.

Getting started

However long it's been, or however unfit you are, you can take the first step and commit yourself to becoming more active. The body never forgets how to adapt positively to exercise, even after several years of inactivity. Start by completing the physical activity readiness questionnaire (PAR-Q) below.

PAR-Q and You (A Questionnaire for People Aged 15 to 69)[5]

Regular physical activity is fun and healthy, and increasingly more people are starting to become more active every day. Being more active is very safe for most people. However, some people should check with their doctor before they start becoming much more physically active.

If you are planning to become much more physically active than you are now, start by answering the seven questions in the box below. If you are between the ages of 15 and 69, the PAR-Q will tell you if you should check with your doctor before you start. If you are over 69 years of age, and you are not used to being very active, check with your doctor.

Common sense is your best guide when you answer these questions. Please read the questions carefully and answer each one honestly: check YES or NO.

Has your doctor ever said that you have a heart condition and that you should only do physical activity recommended by them?

Yes ❏ No ❏

Do you feel pain in your chest when you do physical activity?

Yes ❏ No ❏

In the past month have you had chest pain when you were not doing physical activity?

Yes ❏ No ❏

Do you lose your balance because of dizziness or do you ever lose consciousness?

Yes ❏ No ❏

Do you have a bone or joint problem (e.g. back, knee or hip) that could be made worse by a change in your physical activity?

Yes ❏ No ❏

Is your doctor currently prescribing drugs (for example, water pills) for your blood pressure or heart condition?

Yes ❏ No ❏

Do you know of any other reason why you should not do physical activity?

Yes ❏ No ❏

If you answered 'yes' to one or more questions

Talk to your doctor by phone or in person BEFORE you start becoming much more active or BEFORE you have a fitness appraisal. Tell your doctor about the PAR-Q and to which questions you answered 'yes'.

▶ You may be able to do any activity you want as long as you start slowly and build up gradually. Or, you may need to restrict your activities to those which are safe for you.

▶ Talk to your doctor about the kinds of activities you wish to participate in and follow his/her advice.

If you answered 'no' to PAR-Q questions, you can be reasonably sure that you can:

▶ Start becoming much more physically active – begin slowly and build up gradually. This is the safest and easiest way.

▶ Take part in a fitness appraisal – this is an excellent way to determine your basic fitness. It is also highly recommended that you have your blood pressure evaluated. If your reading is over 144/94, talk with your doctor before you start becoming much more physically active.

Delay becoming much more active:

▶ If you are not feeling well because of a temporary illness such as a cold or a fever – wait until you feel better.

▶ If you are or may be pregnant – talk to your doctor before you start becoming more active.

PLEASE NOTE: If your health changes so that you then answer YES to any of the above questions, tell your fitness or health professional. Ask whether you should change your physical activity plan.

Get more active

Doing more in your daily life – walking rather than driving, taking the stairs rather than the lift – will help burn more calories. Just standing up and moving around is better than sitting. Scientists now think that even if you exercise regularly, too much sitting can negatively affect your health, increasing the risk of type 2 diabetes and heart disease[6], while just getting up and moving around for two minutes every 20 minutes will help reduce that risk[7]. So on top of your planned exercise, aim to increase the amount of other activity you do during the day and to do it more energetically. Lots of little bits of exercise add up and help to increase your total calorie burn. Being active during the day can burn more calories than a single gym session. For ideas on how to include more physical activity in your daily routine see Appendix F, page 338.

What type of exercise?

For weight loss you need to combine:

▶ Cardiovascular (aerobic) exercise – such as brisk walking, cycling or swimming, which raises your heart rate and makes you feel warm and slightly out of breath.

▶ Resistance exercise – using light weights, resistance bands or your own body weight to work your muscles.

Cardiovascular exercise

This type of exercise will help to burn calories and improve your fitness. It lowers your risk of heart disease and some cancers, helps lower blood pressure, improves cholesterol levels, burns off body fat and is a great antidote to stress. Weight-bearing exercise, when we're on our feet walking and running, is important for maintaining bone density, reducing fracture risk as we age.

> *'If I have spent an hour at aerobics burning off 350 kcal, the last thing I want to do is replace it all with 350 kcal of snacks. Thinking about it, you can eat 350 kcal of chocolate or crisps in just minutes.'* Angela, 35

Resistance exercise

This will increase your muscle mass and improve its strength and endurance. More muscle means that your metabolic rate will be higher so that you burn more calories even at rest and your body will become more toned. Resistance work can also help lower blood pressure and cholesterol and improve insulin sensitivity. It's also important for maintaining strong bones and helping maintain healthy joints as the muscles supporting those joints strengthen and provide more support. Stronger muscles also mean a lower risk of falls and injuries and will help to improve your balance.

Flexibility exercise

This is another vital, but often overlooked, part of over- all fitness. Flexibility tends to decline as you get older, but it's vital for everyday life – you can't do simple things like tie your shoelaces or scrub your back in the bath if you have lost flexibility. Flexibility is specific to each joint or set of joints and refers to the maximum range of movement around that joint. If you stretch regularly as part of your fitness programme you will maintain and improve your flexibility. Maintaining flexibility helps to reduce the risk of injury while you are exercising.

Your exercise targets

In the short term (the first six months) you are aiming to build up to 150 minutes' moderate or 75 minutes' vigorous cardio-vascular exercise per week. Vigorous activity will raise your heart rate higher and burn more calories than moderate exercise. This amount of exercise can feel daunting if you're not used to it, so build up to it gradually. You can break it down into shorter sessions and still receive significant health benefits. You may have heard about recent research suggesting that you only need to exercise at high intensity for a few minutes each week. While this has been shown to have some health benefits it won't have a major impact on your weight. To ensure that The 2-Day Diet works most effectively you need to exercise for the recommended amount each week.

Moderate exercise Burns 3–5 times as many calories as many being at rest	Vigorous exercise Burns at least six times as calories as being at rest
Walking at 4–6.4 kph (2½–4 mph)	Fast walking (7.2 kph/4½ mph or 6.4 kph/4 mph uphill) or jog (6.4 kph/4 mph) or quicker
Mowing the lawn	Chopping wood
Badminton	Squash
Ballroom dancing	High-impact aerobics
Leisurely cycling at 9.6 kph (6 mph)	Faster cycling (16 kph/10 mph)
Recreational swimming at a leisurely pace	Swimming (10 lengths of a 25 m/82 ft pool in 5 minutes – any stroke)

You can break your exercise into five shorter sessions (5 x 30 minutes moderate or 5 x 15 minutes vigorous) or do longer sessions less frequently. (This does not include any warm-up or cool-down exercises). If you decide on longer sessions, try to exercise three times a week, since some important health benefits (e.g. cholesterol reduction) only last for 48 hours after exercise. You can combine moderate and vigorous exercise and vary your exercise levels from day to day according to your schedule – on a busy day, for example, you may only manage a 15-minute jog, while another day you might have time to swim for an hour.

In the longer term (six months after starting exercising) you should aim to do 300 minutes of moderate or 150 minutes of vigorous exercise a week because this is the level at which the exercise will help you to lose weight, keep it off and obtain additional health benefits[8].

As well as your cardiovascular exercise, aim to fit in two to three muscle-strengthening resistance exercise sessions each week and two to three flexibility sessions, to reduce the risk of injury and stay as mobile as possible. Although this might sound daunting, you can combine the sessions. Stretch by doing a warm-up and cool-down every time you exercise and add some resistance training to your programme a couple of times a week.

On your marks...

Think carefully about what you want to achieve – and, more importantly, what is realistic for you. Exercise should be achievable, enjoyable, affordable and fit in with your lifestyle and any physical conditions you may have.

Which exercise is best for me?

If you're a complete beginner, you can't go wrong with walking – it's the best free exercise programme there is. For anyone with joint or respiratory problems, swimming provides a whole-body workout, although it's not weight-bearing and won't help maintain healthy bones. Cycling is another non-weight-bearing exercise that's good for joints. Recumbent bikes, where your thighs are in a forward position at 90 degrees to your body, are better for people with back or shoulder problems. Running or jogging is a great free activity, but it can strain your knee and hip joints, especially if you run on hard surfaces – you need to wear good-quality trainers to protect your joints. If you find it hard to stay motivated, exercise classes provide variety, a great social environment and are good for beginners. If you feel too self-conscious to join a class or put on a swimming costume, invest in an exercise DVD or start by borrowing one from the library. Try to find the approach that suits you.

'Feeling trimmer encourages me to exercise and makes me more positive.' Lorna, 53

Wherever you start, the key is to commit yourself. Like you, most regular exercisers have busy lives. The difference is that they make exercise a priority. It takes around three months to form an exercise habit, so schedule it into your life. Look at what you can clear from your diary or identify any spare time you can use to fit in some activity and consider dropping some inactivity (like watching TV) so that you can fit your exercise in.

Choose the time of day that suits you best. Exercising early in the day will help to elevate your mood and energy levels for the day. It's important to warm up properly as your body temperature is lower in the morning, which can increase the risk of injury. When you exercise in the afternoon or evening you tend to put in more effort since exercise feels easier and your muscles are warm.

Exercising out of doors has added benefits, particularly in the summer months when exposure to sunshine will increase your production of vitamin D (winter UV is not strong enough).

Get set....

As with your weight loss, setting yourself some short- and longer-term exercise goals gives you a clear idea of what you're aiming for and helps you track your progress.

▶ **Be specific.** Experts agree that successful exercisers are the ones who set specific goals – just deciding to 'get fit' or 'do more walking' are not specific enough and won't get done. Try to set goals for specific activities with a distance and a time to achieve it in. You might want to set short-term goals such as being able to walk to the shops and back without being out of breath or being able to play a short game of football with your grandchildren. For the longer term you will want to aim at something more ambitious, such as setting yourself a 12-week challenge to build up to swim 30 lengths or walk 10 km (6 miles) or even do a 5 or 10 km (3 or 6 mile) charity run.

▶ **Make it achievable.** Be ambitious but realistic. You can always revise your goals if you reach your target very quickly.

▶ **Give yourself deadlines.** Make sure you give yourself a realistic timeframe to achieve your goal. You may want to break your goal down into more manageable weekly targets.

▶ **Write yourself a contract.** Write down what you want to achieve and why, how you plan to do it and how other people can help. Make copies of your contract and pin them up around your home. Think about creating a blog or a Facebook post saying what you are aiming for and how you plan to achieve it. Once others know about your plans, it will make it harder to give up, and you'll get other people on board to encourage you.

▶ **Schedule your exercise.** Book exercise appointments with yourself in your diary or calendar and stick to them; get up 30 minutes earlier, swap 30 minutes of TV for exercise, or get (or borrow) a dog to walk!

Stay safe

▶ Build up your exercise programme slowly to reduce the likelihood of injuries.

▶ Wear loose, comfortable clothing and choose the right footwear with a good arch support – especially if you are walking or running.

▶ Warm up gently before exercising and cool down slowly afterwards to help prevent injury and help your body adapt and recover (see below).

▶ Always do your stretches on starting and finishing your training.

▶ Don't overexert yourself; signs of overexertion include nausea, sickness, dizziness, light-headedness and chest pain.

▶ Don't exercise outside if the weather is too hot or cold or you are unwell.

▶ Don't eat a big meal before exercise – wait at least one hour after eating before exercising.

▶ Drink plenty of water.

Warm-up

Preparing your joints for exercise helps to reduce the wear and tear on them. You can do these mobilising exercises while you march on the spot – to get your heart rate up and prepare your body for activity. Be aware of your posture as you begin to exercise and try to maintain good posture while exercising. Stand tall and slightly draw the stomach muscles towards the spine to engage the abdominal muscles. Looking forward, relax the shoulders down and try to make them straight by drawing the shoulder blades together. Place feet hip-width apart. Knees should not be locked straight but relaxed and have a slight bend. It's important to complete movements in a gentle, smooth manner, not forcing the joints and pushing them beyond the point where it feels uncomfortable. Repeat each mobility exercise six to ten times.

Joint	Mobility exercise	Description
Head/ neck	Neck tilt	Tilt your head, sending the ear towards your left shoulder, back to the central position and then to your right shoulder
	Neck turn	Turn your head, looking as far left as you can turn it, back to the middle and then look as far right as you can.
	Chin retraction	Draw your head backwards without tilting your chin down, as if you're trying to make a double chin.
Shoulders	Shoulder shrug	Raise your shoulders up towards the ears and then relax back down.
	Shoulder roll	With arms by the sides, roll your shoulders in circles, starting by raising your shoulders towards your ears, then taking them back, down and round in a circle.
	Arm circles	Progress from the shoulder roll by placing your hands on your shoulders and then making circles as if drawing circles with your elbows. Then extend the arm so that it's straight and continue the circling. If it feels uncomfortable, try one arm at a time.

Thoracic spine (upper back)	Torso twist	Keeping your hips facing forward, rotate only the upper part of the body, so that your shoulders and head are in line twisting first left and then right.
Lumbar spine (lower back)	Side bend	Try to remain as straight as possible, as if suspended between two panes of glass. Keep both feet on the floor and tilt your whole body, first to the left and then to the right.
Lumbar spine and hips	Hip circles	Take your hips around in a circle, first clockwise and then anticlockwise.
Knee and hip	Knee to hip	Raise your left leg in front, with the knee bent until it reaches hip height. Repeat with right.
Ankle	Foot point forward and back	Without placing any weight on your leg, point the toes away from your body and then point them back to your body while pushing the heel away.

Pre-exercise stretches

Stretching helps prepare your warmed muscles for further exercise and reduce the risk of injury. Hold each stretch for 10 to 15 seconds on each side.

Calf (Gastrocnemius)

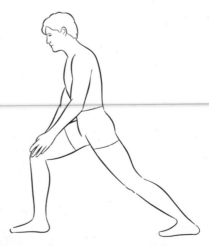

In a standing position, take a step forward and place your right foot out in front, in line with your hips. Your left leg remains outstretched behind you. Lean gently forwards, placing your hands on your right knee for support. You should feel the stretch at the

131

top of your left calf. Try to keep your feet facing forwards and parallel. Don't let the heel on the left leg that's behind you turn inwards.

Back of thigh (Hamstring)

In a standing position take a small step forwards with your right leg. Keep this leg straight and outstretched in front of you, while gently bending your left leg (as though you're squatting) and pushing your bottom backwards. You should feel this stretch in the top of the back of your leg. You can place your hands on your bent knee for support.

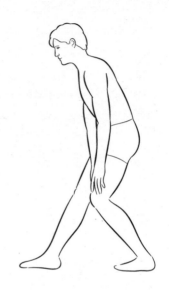

Front of thigh (Quadriceps)

Stand near a wall for support. Bring the heel of your right foot back up towards your buttocks. Hold it with one arm (you can use the other to balance yourself). You should feel this stretch down the front of your thigh. If not, gently tilt your pelvis forwards until you feel the stretch.

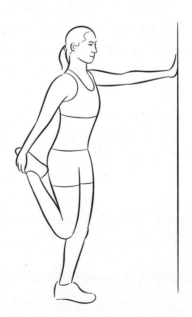

Side (Lats and obliques)

In a standing position, with your feet facing forwards in line with your hips, place your right hand on your right hip and lift your left arm up along your side and over your head. At the same time, lean to your right. You should feel the stretch from under your arm all the way down the left side of your torso.

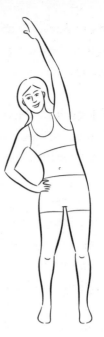

Shoulder

In a standing position, place your right arm across your body, making sure not to lock your elbow. Then use your left arm and place your hand on your upper arm and gently pull your right arm in towards your body.

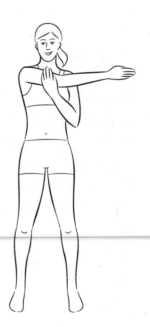

Back of arm (Triceps)

In a standing position, raise one arm straight above your head. Bend the elbow so that your hand is reach- ing down to touch the back of your shoulder. Use the other hand to support the raised arm.

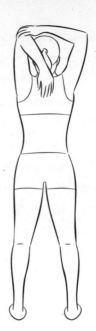

Shoulder (Pectorals and deltoid)

Standing side on to the wall place your right palm against it. Take one or two steps forwards, keeping your palm flat against the wall. Allow your palm to turn, so your fingers are pointing in the opposite direction. Allow your body to twist slightly to the left. You should feel the stretch in your shoulder and across your chest.

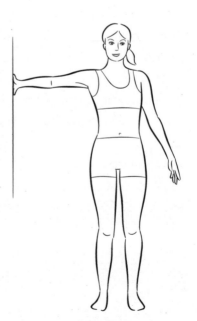

Cool-down

Slow down gradually, over four to six minutes, to help your heart rate and breathing return to normal. If you stop suddenly, without cooling down, it can leave you feeling dizzy, sick or faint. As you get fitter your body will respond more readily to changes in physical exertion and your heart rate will return to normal more quickly. Repeat your warm-up stretches, but this time hold them for up to 60 seconds to help improve your flexibility and prevent stiffness.

Cardiovascular exercise

If you're a complete beginner walking is, without doubt, the cheapest, easiest and safest way to get fit. Start gently and aim to walk at a pace that is comfortable for you, but which makes you feel slightly warm and slightly out of breath, but still able to talk. Plan a route that is circular, safe, preferably flat, and ideally interesting. Don't worry too much about the distance – as you become fitter you will be able to walk further in the same time. Walking is a very safe form of exercise, so you won't necessarily need to warm up unless you're doing morning walks or longer, faster walks.

We've designed a 12-week programme so you can build up over the weeks. If the first week feels too easy, start at the level of week three or four. If you're struggling repeat a week until you're ready to move on. You must complete the full 12 weeks. By your twelfth week you should be doing 150 minutes' moderate exercise – that's about half an hour for five days a week – wherever you were at the start. For your 12-week walking plan see Appendix G, page 339.

Monitor your cardiovascular progress

It is important to monitor yourself, to ensure that you are exercising at the right intensity and that you are exercising safely.

The Talk Test is a simple way to check that you're working at the right level. You should be a little breathless, but still able to hold a conversation. If you're struggling to talk in sentences, you're overdoing it and need to slow down.

The Rate of Perceived Exertion (RPE) is a numerical scale from 1 to 10 (with 1 being the lowest intensity and 10 the highest) that you can use while exercising to gauge how you are feeling and know whether you need to speed up or slow down to get you training at the right intensity.

- ▶ 0 = No exertion at all
- ▶ 1 = Very, very light exertion
- ▶ 2 = Very light exertion
- ▶ 3 = Light exertion
- ▶ 4 = Moderate exertion
- ▶ 5 = Somewhat hard (you need to make an effort to maintain a conversation)
- ▶ 6 = Hard
- ▶ 7 = Very hard
- ▶ 8 = Very, very hard
- ▶ 9 = Extremely hard
- ▶ 10 = Absolute maximal effort (no conversation is possible and breathing is very hard)

You'll get the most benefits from exercise when you are working at least at a moderate intensity (4 to 5 on the scale). You should feel slightly warm and be breathing more heavily, but still be able to talk. Try to maintain this level for the exercise period – if it gets too easy pick up the pace. If you are struggling, tone the pace down. Practise using the system while walking before you try it in other exercise situations. As well as keeping you on track, it will help you to monitor your progress – as you get fitter you may find that you score the same walk or run a 3 instead of a 4.

Resistance exercise

You are aiming to increase your amount of body muscle as well as the endurance and strength of your muscles. For endurance training you need a lighter weight or smaller resistance and more repetitions. For strength training you need a heavier weight or greater resistance and fewer repetitions.

We've designed the resistance sessions to work for everyone, whatever their fitness level. Do them two to three times a week to help maintain your muscle mass while you're losing weight. Always do a warm-up and cool-down before and after resistance training.

▶ Keep your movements slow and controlled, both when you contract and relax the muscle.

▶ Focus on your breathing – you should breathe out on exertion and breathe in as you relax the muscle. As with the stretches, avoid holding your breath when you're concentrating on an exercise.

▶ Think about your posture and balance. Stand in front of a mirror to check your posture. Stand tall – imagine a string attached to the top of your head pulling upwards – with your shoulders relaxed and down and your weight balanced equally on each foot, with your feet hip-width apart. Good posture will help the important core muscles around your back and stomach area to do their job properly.

▶ These exercises shouldn't hurt or be uncomfortable – if they are, stop!

▶ Avoid locking your elbows or knees straight or over-extending joints.

▶ Familiarise yourself with the jargon. Exercise programmes often refer to 'sets' and 'reps' (repetitions), so 'one set of 10 reps' for a bicep curl would be 10 repetitions of a bicep curl and two sets of 10 reps would be 10 repetitions, a pause or rest and then another 10 repetitions.

You can do repetitive resistance exercises using free weights (dumbbells), resistance bands, the weight of your own body, inflatable gym balls or one of the many different exer- cise gadgets on the market. Free weights don't have to cost you a penny. Water weighs 1 g per ml so if you fill a 500 ml (17½ fl oz) plastic water bottle your handmade weight will be
500 g (1 lb 1 oz). To make heavier weights, fill bottles with sand. Once you start needing heavier weights you might want to think about buying a set. Latex resistance bands come in a variety of colours, which refer to their thickness. The thicker they are, the tougher they are to stretch and the more resist- ance they produce. They can be used with most exercises: for example, to do bicep curls, place the resistance band on the floor and position your foot in the middle of the band. Pick up an end of the band in either hand, making sure you have a good grip. You can then use the resistance of the band to do your bicep curls. Don't wrap the band around your hand and cut off the blood flow. If you're using your own body weight for a resistance exercise, for example a press-up/push-up, make sure you start with the easiest position before you progress over time: for example, start by pressing from all fours and progress to full-on toes press-ups.

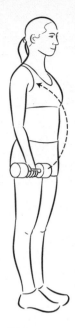

Bicep curls

Active muscles: Biceps

Description: Stand with your feet shoulder-width apart and your arms down by your sides, palms facing forwards. With a light weight in your right hand, bring the weight up towards the shoulder. Bend the elbow but keep it by your side. Switch arms and repeat.

Progression: 1. Try doing both arms together.
2. Increase the weight.

Triceps extension

Active muscles: Triceps

Description: Lying on the floor on your back with a light weight in your right hand, raise it straight above your head, gently bending your elbow, lowering the weight to the side of your head. Switch arms and repeat.

Progression: 1. Try doing both arms together.
2. Increase the weight.
3. Do the exercise standing up allowing the arm and weight to go behind the head.

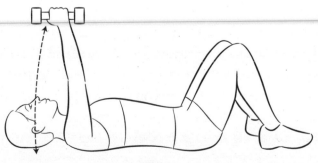

Push-ups

Active muscles: Chest (Pectoral muscles)

Description: Kneeling on all-fours, with your hands flat on the floor shoulder-width apart, lift your feet off the floor so that the weight is now on your knees and arms. Slowly bend your elbows, keeping your back straight, taking your nose to the ground.

Progression: 1. Extend your legs, going up onto your toes, spreading your legs apart and repeat.

2. Extend your legs, going up onto your toes and keep your feet together.

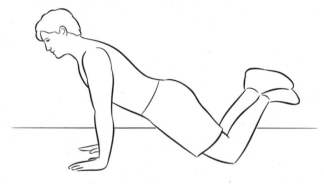

Plank

Active muscles: Abdominals

Description: Lying on your front with palms and all of your lower arm in contact with the floor, think of yourself from neck to toes as one long, rigid piece of wood. Raise yourself up (the palm and lower arm stay in contact with the floor) and you're on your toes in a position similar to a press-up but much closer to the floor. Hold this straight, horizontal plank position. Be very careful if you suffer from lower-back problems. Try not to cave in and let your stomach fall to the floor. If the plank feels too intense, relax to the floor and try an easier version on all-fours. Progress by moving your knee position further back, until your legs are straight as above.

Progression: 1. While you are in the plank position, raise one leg 2.5 cm (1 in) off the ground, hold for two seconds and switch legs.

2. Rotate to the side so that your elbow, shoulder and head are in a line.

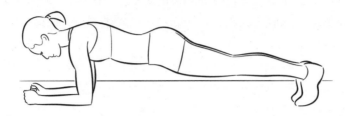

Single arm row

Active muscles: Back and biceps

Description: Stand with your feet shoulder-width apart, legs and back straight. Lean forwards holding a weight in one hand and, arm extended, pull the weight back towards you, bending the elbow. Repeat with the other arm.

Progression: 1. Exercise both arms together.

2. Increase weight.

3. Lean over further (make sure your back is straight).

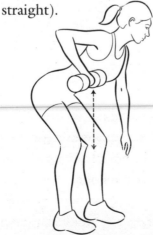

Squats

Active muscles: Thighs and buttocks (Hamstrings, quadriceps and gluteal muscles)

Description: Stand with your feet slightly wider than hip distance apart, with both feet facing forwards. Slowly push your bum backwards and then, keeping a straight back, shoulders and your head up, bend at the knees, in a sitting motion.

Progression: 1. Raise your arms up straight as you squat.

                2. Try the same thing, but with small weights.

                3. Try while doing arm weights (e.g. bicep curls).

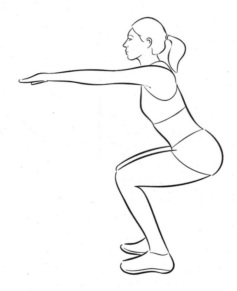

Home circuit class

For a complete workout, combine cardiovascular, resistance and flexibility training, and make yourself a home circuit using five or six of the above resistance exercises. Alternate between leg and arm exercises to prevent fatigue and add marching, side-stepping or skipping in between each strengthening exercise to raise your heart rate. Start with low, or no, weights and slowly increase as you progress. Gradually add more exercises to your circuit and increase the number of repetitions and sets that you do. Cool down and stretch to complete your workout. The exercises that you can do with weights are marked * in the table.

'I have enjoyed getting into clothes that haven't fitted for a long time and I'm really feeling the benefits of increased fitness from exercise.' Sam, 29

Exercise	Week 1	Week 4	Week 8
Squat	1 set x 10 reps	2 sets x 10 reps	3 sets x 10 reps
Bicep curls*	1 set x 10 reps	2 sets x 10 reps	3 sets x 10 reps
Lunges	1 set x 10 reps	2 sets x 10 reps	3 sets x 10 reps
Triceps extensions*	1 set x 10 reps	2 sets x 10 reps	3 sets x 10 reps
Plank	2 sets 20 second holds	2 sets 30 second holds	3 sets 40 second holds
Push-ups	1 set x 10 reps	2 sets x 10 reps	3 sets x 10 reps

After the first 12 weeks ...

You can continue with the same exercise programme for the next three months, to give your body time to adapt before you step things up to aim for 300 minutes of moderate or 150 minutes' vigorous cardiovascular exercise a week. If you feel ready to do more before the end of the three months, go for it! Remember that you don't have to stick with the same exercise classes or activity, but you should keep doing the same amount of exercise, at the same level of intensity.

For more exercise ideas beyond the first 12 weeks and information on exercise targets see our website (www.thetwodaydiet. co.uk).

How to stay motivated

Vary your routine

Change what you do every six to eight weeks to avoid getting bored and reaching a plateau in your fitness. If you keep doing the same exercise your body will adapt to it, so that it is no longer challenging and your fitness won't improve. For example, if you're walking, include some hills or find a new route; if you are swimming, vary your strokes, or add a completely different type of exercise to your weekly schedule. If you're a gym member, ask your instructor to design you a new programme every three months.

Find a new challenge

Learning a new skill is always empowering, so if you are feeling more body-confident now why not learn to dance? Ballroom dancing is not just for the celebrities. Alternatively, why not revisit a sport you used to play – perhaps one you were keen on in your school days? Perhaps you used to play tennis but stopped? Find a local club for new people to play with.

Measure yourself

Waist, hips and bust are the most obvious parts of the body to measure, but you might want to keep track of your upper arm or thigh measurements. Measure your waist to see whether you're losing abdominal fat (see page 33).

Record the changes

The camera never lies so why not keep 'before' and 'after' pictures pinned up on your fridge to help keep you on track and focused on your exercise regime. Visible evidence of the way your body is changing will help to encourage you to persevere.

Just do a little

When you feel pushed for time or really demotivated just try to do 10 minutes of activity. You're getting some health benefits and you might find that by committing to doing 10 minutes of exercise you end up doing more.

Be flexible

If your exercise bike breaks, don't give up until it's fixed: try something different. If you have less time one week to fit in your exercise sessions try to exercise harder for less time. Life tends to throw lots of things at us and we can't let it derail our good intentions.

Monitor your workouts

If you feel the frequency of your workouts might be slipping, use apps or a simple diary to monitor yourself and to remind you to exercise.

Sign up

Try entering a sponsored swim, run or bike ride. Alternatively sponsor yourself and give a donation to charity when you have achieved a personal fitness goal.

Adapt your exercise programme

If you know you're heading towards a busy month or if you feel your time commitment to exercise is wavering, think about changing your approach and focus on intensity rather than frequency. If you've been exercising at a moderate level, increase the intensity of your workout to a vigorous level and decrease the frequency of your workouts. This way, you're meeting the recommended exercise guidelines in literally half the time.

Reward yourself

Set yourself mini goals every couple of weeks – to walk further, faster, add five minutes to your routine – and give yourself a reward (that's not food or alcohol) when you achieve your goal.

Your questions answered

'How will I know if I'm getting fitter?'

Take your resting pulse rate. Sit down for five minutes (10 if you've been active). Then place two fingers on the inside of your wrist and count the number of pulse beats in a minute. Do this weekly – as you get fitter, your pulse rate will get slower.

Do a simple walking/running test. Walk or run a mile. Time how long it takes you, measure your pulse at the end and score your RPE (see page 136). Repeat the test after 12 weeks.

'Will exercise make me hungry?'

We all react differently to increasing our activity levels – half of us naturally eat more, the other half either eat less or roughly the same amount[9]. As you step up your exercise, monitor your eating and make sure you don't reward yourself or 'compensate' for exercise done by having larger servings or 'treats' of high-sugar, high-fat foods.

Exercise is actually well known for helping to regulate your appetite and doing some activity on restricted days could help to distract you and stop you getting bored, especially in the evenings when you might be tempted to break your diet.

'Should I have a sports drink to keep my energy levels up?'

Staying well hydrated while exercising is vital for your energy levels and your overall health, but water is the best thing to drink. A 500 ml (17½ fl oz) sports drink contains between 150 and 350 calories, most of it sugar. Ignore the marketing hype – unless you're an elite athlete in training you're unlikely to need anything more than water.

'How many calories will I burn?'

It's tempting to think that if you're exercising you can eat what you like – in fact, as you can see below, it takes a lot of exercise to burn off even a small amount of food. The number of calories burnt has been estimated for a woman weighing 11 stone (70 kg)[10]. If you are heavier than this you will burn off slightly more calories during each activity; if you are lighter you will burn off slightly fewer.

Half an hour of…	Calories burnt by an 11 stone (70 kg) woman	Examples of food burnt off
Hoovering	115	300 ml (10 fl oz) of orange juice 4 thin mint fondant-filled chocolates 3 wrapped chocolates
Gardening moderate effort	122	A 25 g (¾ oz) bag of crisps A 250 ml (8½ fl oz) bottle of fruit smoothie A 125 g (41/3 oz) pot of whole milk yoghurt
Walking 3.5 mph (5.6 kph)	150	A 40 g (1½ oz) fondant-filled chocolate egg 284 ml (½ pint) lager 35 g (1¼ oz) Cheddar cheese
Aerobics: low impact	175	2 chocolate digestive biscuits A 175 ml (6 fl oz) glass of wine A 60 g (2 oz) scoop luxury ice cream
Swimming: Breaststroke, light recreational	185	A small bottle (380 ml/13 fl oz) of energy drink 3 plain digestive biscuits A 30 g (1 oz) bag of crisps

Half an hour of...	Calories burnt by an 11 stone (70 kg) woman	Examples of food burnt off
Cycling 9 mph (14.5 kph)	203	Half a cheese sandwich A tube of fruit pastilles A large latte coffee
Aerobics: high impact	255	A 250 ml (8½ fl oz) glass of wine A 440 ml (15½ fl oz) can of lager 50 g (1¾ oz) of milk chocolate
Jogging 5 mph (8 kph)	290	200 g (7 oz) chicken chow mein (takeaway) 500 ml (17½ fl oz) cola Half a double burger (108 g/3½ oz) (fast food outlet)
Running 7 mph (11 kph)	384	200 g (7 oz) egg fried rice (takeaway) 117 g (4 oz) medium serving French fries A fast food medium strawberry milk shake

'Can I spot-reduce problem areas like my bottom and waist?'

Although there's no evidence that you can spot-reduce fat by spending a lot of time exercising specific areas, what does seem clear is that you tend to lose fat more quickly from some areas of the body than others when you lose weight and do exercise. Getting your recommended 150–300 minutes of moder- ate cardiovascular exercise – doing things like brisk walking or jogging – can boost the loss of unhealthy intra-abdominal fat, which should both improve your health and reduce your waist measurement[11]. And although we still don't have conclusive evidence, we think that the two strict days of dieting each week with The 2-Day Diet could have a greater impact on abdominal fat. Exercise will also tone muscles, helping you to feel more toned in areas such as your bottom, thighs and tummy.

'Can I exercise on restricted days of the diet?'

Lots of people think that because they are limiting calories, and particularly carbs, they won't have the energy to exercise on the restricted two days of The 2-Day Diet. In fact we found that this wasn't the case. Our Dieters were just as likely to exercise on the two restricted as the five unrestric- ted days and the calorie and carbohydrate restrictions didn't seem to reduce their ability to exercise or increase their levels of fatigue. Some of the Dieters actually recorded 60 minutes of vigorous activity and as much as four hours of moderate activity on restricted days of the diet. Other research bears out the fact that your exercise capacity and tolerance shouldn't dip on restricted days[12] – in fact one study suggested that if you are doing a low-carb, low-calorie diet you might burn more fat while exercising than if you were following a high-carb, low-cal diet. Make sure you stay well hydrated and get your sodium, potassium and permitted 50 g of carbohydrates in your dairy, fruit and vegetable allowance.

If you are normally a vigorous exerciser and are struggling with this on your two restricted days of The 2-Day Diet, we recommend replacing vigorous with moderate activity and save the vigorous workouts for your unrestricted days.

'Is it better to exercise before breakfast or when I haven't eaten for a while, or to exercise after meals?'

When you exercise, your body takes energy from carbohydrates, or if they're not available, from burning your fat stores. A question that has intrigued sports scientists is whether exercising when you haven't eaten for a while – in other words when there is no available carbohydrate energy – can boost the amount of fat you burn. A recent study suggests that this may be the case. In a very carefully controlled exper- iment, researchers in Glasgow asked 10 overweight and normally sedentary men to walk for an hour either immedi- ately before or immediately after a 450-calorie breakfast. They then moni- tored how much fat was burned off during the exercise and for eight and a half hours afterwards. Although both exer- cise sessions burnt fat, the men who exercised before breakfast burnt 40 per cent more fat than those who walked after eating[13]. So although exercising at any time will help with your weight loss, you may get an extra boost from doing it before, rather than soon after, meals.

Using a pedometer

A pedometer is a great way to track your walking progress or to measure how much more activity you're clocking up in a normal day. We should all be aiming for between 7,000 and 11,000 steps per day, at least 3,000 should be done at a brisk pace.

Pedometers work by sensing the force your body generates when you take a step. You clip them onto your waistband and they tot up your steps as you get on with your life. Because they sense force, be aware that they can also record non-walking activities such as going over a speed bump when driving! Avoid the cheapest machines, which can be unreliable, and go for a mid-range model. Make sure your pedometer does not slip or turn during walking or it may not record correctly.

To check that a new pedometer is measuring accurately, walk 50 steps. If it is not correct ensure that it is vertical on your hip and move it around until you find the place to wear it, where it will give you an accurate count. Some pedometers are worn as watches or carried in a pocket, but again, try to test them for accuracy. Some pedometers provide you with an estimate of calories burned and distance covered. It is important to remember that these estimates are not tailored to you and so are not a reliable measure. If you want to measure calories burned look for a pedometer that allows you to input your weight, height, gender, and stride length if you want to know the distance you are covering. Some companies have designed pedometers that can link to your phone or MP3 player (sometimes worn as an armband or on trainers) and some can be linked to your computer so you can download your daily steps and track your progress.

Dealing with problems

Aching muscles

Don't be surprised if your muscles protest a bit at first – you'll find you will probably ache most 48 hours after exercising! It will get better. Doing a proper warm-up and cool-down is thought to decrease the risk of injury, especially if you are not used to exercise.

Dehydration

Stay hydrated. Drink water rather than sports drinks, which tend to be loaded with sugar and calories. If you've had a particularly sweaty workout try a small glass of skimmed milk to replenish your electrolyte and sugar levels.

Joint pain

Muscle-strengthening exercises, Pilates or yoga will help strengthen muscles supporting your joints and should help with knee and hip pain, but if you have achy joints you should see your GP. Although the evidence is limited, you might want to try Glucosamine and/or Chondroitin Sulphate. There's some evidence that a daily 1,500 mg glucosamine supplement can provide modest pain relief for some people. The MHRA (Medicines and Healthcare Regulatory Authority) has warned against its use by people who have seafood allergies or those who are taking Warfarin. Check with your GP before taking any health dietary supplement.

Fatigue

Exercise can make you feel a little tired, but if you need to sit down for more than 30 minutes afterwards, you're overdoing it and you need to slow down. Try reducing the frequency and the intensity of the exercise and see how you feel next time.

Injury

If you build up exercise gradually at your own pace you shouldn't get injured but if you do, see your GP and physio-therapist and take their advice about how quickly to return to exercising. Rehabilitation exercise, such as swimming (after receiving the okay from your GP), is an easy and supportive form of exercise to get you back into the swing of things.

Should I buy a heart rate monitor?

You don't need to buy one, but if you fancy the idea of having a gadget that can tell you whether you are working hard enough and help monitor your progress you might want to invest in a basic monitor (priced around £15–£20) and you can upgrade as you progress. Some are like watches, which take your thumb pulse when placed on the screen; others use separate chest straps that register and transmit your heart rate to a watch every few seconds. You can also download a heart rate monitor as an app to your mobile phone. Using heart rate zones allows you to exercise safely at different intensities. Your maximum heart rate (in beats per minute) is 220 minus your age, so if you are 40, it will be 180 beats per minute.

The different heart rate zones, which work in percentages of your maximum heart rate, are:

- Moderate exercise = 50 to 70%
  50–60% of maximum heart rate = Moderate Aerobic Zone
  60–70% of maximum heart rate = Aerobic Weight Management Zone

- Vigorous exercise = 70 to 85%
  70–80% of maximum heart rate = Aerobic Fitness Zone
  80–90% of maximum heart rate = Peak Aerobic Performance Zone

Exercising at a heart rate between 80–90% of maximum heart rate is only suitable for trained individuals.

Summary

▶ Regular exercise will enhance the benefits of The 2-Day Diet by burning calories and maintaining calorie-burning muscle. It also helps protect against heart disease, type 2 diabetes and many cancers and will boost your mood and energy levels.

▶ Before starting an exercise programme make sure that you are fit enough. If in doubt, see your GP.

▶ To benefit your health you need to do 150 minutes moderate or 75 minutes of vigorous exercise each week. For weight loss and added health benefits you need to build up to 300 minutes of moderate or 150 minutes of vigorous exercise each week.

▶ Aim to do strengthening exercises 2–3 times per week.

▶ Try to do exercises that will improve your flexibility 2 times per week.

▶ It's important to combine cardiovascular exercise with resistance exercises to strengthen your muscles and stretching to improve flexibility.

▶ You can break exercise into smaller or longer chunks and do it every day or less frequently, but ideally at least once every two days.

▶ Ensure that you warm up and cool down properly each time you exercise, to help avoid injury.

▶ Once you get into the exercise habit, set yourself new goals and ring the changes to avoid becoming bored.

7

how to
stay slim

Congratulations! If you are reading this chapter you have probably reached your weight-loss goal with The 2-Day Diet and are ready to move into the next phase: keeping the pounds off and maintaining your fantastic new look and weight. We know that it's taken huge commitment and a lot of hard work to get to this point and you need to give yourself a huge pat on the back for your amazing achievement.

But let's pause here – your work is not yet done! The big temptation for any dieter who has achieved their goal weight is to accept the praise, heave a huge sigh of relief that the diet is over and go back to eating the way they were before starting the diet. And some of you reading this will have been there already – possibly several times – and will know how devastating it feels when you see the weight starting to creep back on.

But don't worry! This chapter will give you the tools you need to make sure that this doesn't happen again. You haven't done all this hard work only to go back to where you started. The vital thing to recognise is that having reached your weight-loss goal is not the end but an important transition time. Like losing weight, *maintaining* the weight you have achieved will take commitment, vigilance and perseverance. It can be just as much of a challenge as getting the weight off in the first place, but this time you are able to build on your success, and use the skills you have acquired along the way and capitalise on the way you have retrained your eating and your exercise habits.

> *'My lapses almost always come when I drink alcohol, for*
> *example after a few glasses of wine on a Friday night.*
> *I do well all week, then after a drink I tend to eat more.*
> *But now I know this I've pretty much cut it out.'*
> Rose, 52

How your body is different

Big changes have taken place in your body since you started The 2-Day Diet. You now weigh less, so your body needs fewer calories for its basic metabolism, upkeep and movement than it did before you started dieting. If you think of this as being like the difference between walking around as you are now and then with a rucksack packed with the weight you have lost, you can appreciate why you needed more energy and calories. Losing weight with any diet also means that many hormones in your body will change, including hormones that increase your appetite and stop you feeling full as quickly[1]. Dieting probably also means that your muscles will have become more efficient and need less energy to function. While this is good news for your muscles, it means that you could now need up to 15 per cent fewer calories than someone of the same weight who hasn't dieted.

The bottom line is that having lost your weight you now need to eat around 400 to 600 fewer calories each day than you did before you started dieting and you must keep exercising to help burn off calories and offset the changes in your metabolism[2]. If you go back to your previous lifestyle you will regain the weight at least as quickly as you lost it.

While all this sounds daunting, we know from our own research that 2-Day Dieters can and do succeed in keeping the weight off. Our first 2-Day Diet study followed up our 2-Day Dieters for 12–15 months. This group had lost around 1½ stone (9.5 kg), going from on average 12 stone 11 lb (81 kg) to 11 stone 5 lb (72 kg) on The 2-Day Diet. They then switched to one restricted day per week to maintain weight loss. After six to nine months of this 1-Day Maintenance Diet they weighed, on average 11 stone 10 lb (74.3 kg) – so had kept off a stone (6.4 kg).

Crucially for their health, one restricted day per week had maintained the beneficial reductions in their blood pressure, cholesterol and insulin. Normally, when you stop following a standard calorie-controlled diet you revert to eating your full calorie requirements on a daily basis. This is when some of the health benefits you've gained from losing weight, particularly the drop in insulin, blood pressure and cholesterol, often start to drift upwards.

How to keep the weight off

So to maintain your weight loss we recommend simply switching to The 1-Day Maintenance Diet as part of our weight-maintenance plan. This plan has been designed in the knowledge that weight maintenance is a new challenge that requires you to keep your calorie intake down and exercise levels up. It requires you to build on the skills you have used for weight loss, but requires a different way of thinking. The section below highlights the dietary guidelines for the one restricted day and six unrestricted Mediterranean diet days. We have also designed an exercise plan to help you keep the weight off (see www.thetwodaydiet.co.uk).

This chapter aims to give you the strategies you need to make sure the weight stays off for good.

'It's harder to follow the diet when you are out in restaurants or at people's houses when they have cooked for you. You have to make sure you tell them in advance.'
Diana, 49

The 1-Day Maintenance Diet

The 1-Day Maintenance Diet is based on The 2-Day Diet, but instead of two restricted days each week you now only have to do one. For the rest of the week (the other six days) we advise you to eat the healthy Mediterranean diet you have followed with the 2-Day Diet (see page 70). Like The 2-Day Diet, you should not have to count calories or weigh food for your 1-Day Maintenance Diet but, as before, make sure that you are keeping within the recommended amounts.

Once again, it's important that on your one restricted day you meet the minimum recommended servings for protein, fruit, vegetables and dairy foods, and don't exceed the maximum recommendations for protein and fats. On the six unrestricted days of The 1-Day Maintenance Diet make sure that you get enough protein, fruit and vegetables, but keep within the maximum amounts. Don't forget, you will need to check the Diet in the Ready Reckoners in Appendix D (see pages 328–336), which tells you the number of servings you can eat on these days for your new lower weight. The Diet has been calculated to account for the fact that you are a successful Dieter and has assumed that your weight has dropped and so your energy requirements are likely to have lowered since you first started The 2-Day Diet.

You may recall that after your two restricted days on The 2-Day Diet your weight dropped partly as a result of losing water. You will also lose water after your one restricted day on The 1-Day Maintenance Diet, so when you weigh yourself, remember to do it just before and not during or immediately after your restricted day.

Adjust your thinking

As well as following a different diet plan you need to adjust your mental approach to put you in the right frame of mind for keeping the weight off permanently.

In some ways, starting a new diet is the easiest part of weight loss. It's new, you're full of hope for the future and you hopefully have the support and encouragement of the people around you who are willing you to succeed. And when you do succeed and the weight comes off, your efforts are constantly rewarded by the compliments you receive about how good you look, and the fact that, at long last, you can start to wear the clothes you like and do the things you enjoy.

Weight maintenance is a completely different ball game. You don't have the excitement of a new challenge and no one is going to marvel and congratulate you about the fact that you are managing to keep the weight off (although they should, because it's a great achievement!). Your challenge now is to make weight control a way of life using the expertise you've gained from mastering The 2-Day Diet.

> *'The times I've not stuck to it have been when I was busy with work, rushing between meetings. It's difficult to control your environment as you are obliged to take what's on offer – I have had to plan for that.'* Theresa, 43

Key tips for maintaining your weight loss

1. Monitor yourself

Keeping a close eye on your weight is a key part of keeping the weight off. If you spot early signs of weight gain you can act quickly and reverse the trend. Weigh yourself weekly, just as you have done throughout The 2-Day Diet, as well as keeping an eye on how your clothes fit – a garment becoming a bit tight could indicate that you are putting on a few pounds. Don't be tempted to 'cheat' by always wearing loose clothing such as joggers or leggings as you're unlikely to notice any change – more snugly fitting clothes are better indicators. If you notice your clothes becoming tighter, weigh yourself. Weight can fluctuate by 2–4½ lb (1–2 kg), but if your weight increases by more than 4½ lb (2 kg) or by 3 per cent of your total weight, this is an alarm bell ringing to tell you to get back on track with your diet and exercise plan.

2. Stay motivated

Revisit your original reasons for wanting to lose weight and remind yourself of how far you have come. You set yourself goals at the start of The 2-Day Diet and it's a really good idea to also set yourself clear targets for keeping the weight off. You might want to keep the weight off for a forthcoming event such as a wedding, a party or a holiday.

We have already mentioned how you can use 'before' dieting pictures to motivate yourself to stay on track when losing weight. You can also use 'before' and 'after' dieting pictures to remind yourself what you have achieved with all your hard work and use this as an incentive for keeping the weight off. Clothes that you can now get into, which you could not before starting to diet, are also a great reminder of how far you have come.

Rewards for achieving your goals – and for sticking with your eating and exercise plan – are even more important when it comes to weight maintenance than for losing weight as you won't have the immediate thrill of seeing the weight coming off. Plan a treat for yourself at the end of each month that you have kept your weight off. In fact, given how challenging it can be, you should probably reward yourself more for weight maintenance than you did for weight loss.

3. Set up your support systems

As well as rewarding yourself, we know there is nothing quite as motivating as receiving positive comments and support from the people around you. This may not automatically happen and so you may need to ask your nearest and dearest for their help. Ask the people who supported you when you were trying to lose weight to carry on with their encouragement as you work at keeping it off. Explain to them that this is an important time for you, with its own challenges. Their support is required to help you keep to your diet plan of one restricted day per week, and an unrestricted Mediterranean diet for six days per week plus your regular exercise plan. Having people to acknowledge your achievements in keeping the weight off is every bit as important as their support for losing weight has been over the months of the diet.

4. Be prepared

The experience of doing The 2-Day Diet will have made you aware of the danger times, which can divert you from your good intentions with eating and exercise. We talked about this in chapters 2 and 5 (see pages 38 and 95), and it might be worth going back to your original list to remind yourself of the strategies that work for you when it comes to fend- ing off temptation or dealing with difficult situations. Use the stress-management strategies to overcome the trap of comfort-eating and plan ahead for social situations. You might decide to allow yourself to eat more freely when it comes to particular social events, but compensate by eating less in the days before and afterwards. If there are occasions when you feel that you have lapsed, don't give up; instead, learn from them to enable you to cope better the next time around.

There can also be longer-term issues that can interfere with weight maintenance. For example, a very busy spell at work when you are stuck in the office until late at night, home improvements, which leave you unable to use your kitchen, periods where you are working away from home and sleeping and eating in hotels can all hamper healthy eating and exercise routines. The good thing is that you can usually see these things looming on the horizon and can plan around them.

'If I do lapse I try to get straight back on track
– I may cut back on something else to balance out
"the transgression".' Heather, 57

CASE STUDY: Annabell

Annabell's story shows just what it's possible to achieve. When Annabell, 35, started our first 2-Day Diet she had a BMI of 38 and weighed almost 14½ stone (92 kg). After 15 months on The 2-Day Diet she lost nearly 3½ stone (22 kg) and five years on she has maintained that weight loss.

'I had tried low-calorie diets before and I'd tried just eating less, but although I always lost a few pounds, I quickly got fed up and stopped. The 2-Day Diet worked for me because it was structured. I found the two restricted days of The 2-Day Diet easy because the rules were so clear and once I reached my goal weight I did The 1-Day Maintenance Diet. I weigh myself once a week, but I can tell by my clothes if I'm gaining weight. I often do one day per week to keep me in check, but I usually gain about 4 lb (1.8 kg) when I go on holiday. Now I just go back onto two days per week of dieting when I get home and it comes back off. Eating like this has become a way of life and I'm still getting positive feedback from family and friends. When I started The 2-Day Diet I was out of breath just walking up stairs; now I regularly do 90-minute brisk walks, play badminton and go to Zumba. It's changed me: I'm more confident, I'm happier, I can wear skirts for the first time in years and I have so much more energy to do things with my daughter.'

5. Watch for portion creep

By the time they completed The 2-Day Diet most of our Dieters had a more realistic idea about the size of a healthy serving of food, but it's still important to keep track of your serving sizes. We're not suggesting that you become obsessive and weigh all of your food, but it's surprisingly easy for servings to get bigger without really noticing it. It helps to use the simple household measures we describe to check your servings. For example, don't just pour out the cereal, rice or pasta, use spoons or a small cup (not a big mug!). It might also help to use smaller plates and bowls and small cutlery. At the end of the day tot up the number of food servings you have had against the recommended amounts for the Diet using the progress charts at www.thetwodaydiet.co.uk.

6. Are you active enough?

Once you reach the maintenance stage you need to be aiming to do 300 minutes' moderate, or 150 minutes' vigorous, exercise spread over the week (see chapter 6). Again, it can be easy to let this slip, so monitor what you do. All the evidence suggests that successful maintainers keep a close eye on their activity levels as well as their weight. You can do a quick mental tally of how active you have been at the end of each day. Write it in a diary or use The 2-Day Diet on-line tool. Don't forget that as you get lighter and fitter you will find exercise easier. Although this is great it does also mean that you won't use as many calories when you exercise as when you first started out. This is why, as you lose weight, you need to keep challenging your body with more demanding workouts.

'When I go out for meals, I simply have reduced servings to enable me to stick to the Diet, as I am never very sure how the food was prepared.' Alicia, 47

7. Keep it varied

Some of us love routine, but if you feel you are stuck in a rut with your diet and exercise, ring the changes. Try different foods and experiment with some of the other recipes in this book (see chapters 9 and 10), not just the four or five favourites you have done so far. Set yourself some different exercise goals, adapt your routine, introduce a different activity to your weekly routine or take up a new challenge such as a half marathon or a charity bike ride.

CASE STUDY: Jane

Jane, 51, has always struggled with her weight. In fact she took part in three previous weight-loss studies at the Genesis Preven- tion Centre and although she was really successful and lost 2–3 stone (12–19 kg) each time, she also put all the weight back on – and sometimes more – once within just five months of reaching her goal weight. But following The 2-Day Diet has been a very different story: weighing in at the beginning of the Diet at just over 17½ stone (111 kg) Jane managed to lose 3 stone (19 kg) within seven months; even more impressive, two and a half years on she has maintained her weight loss and is thrilled with her success.

'I liked The 2-Day Diet right from the beginning because I was able to be really strict with myself on my two restricted diet days and although I was careful during the other days, I didn't feel that I was dieting because it was so different. I lost a lot of weight at first and then it slowed down, but I then joined a gym, which gave me another spurt.

When I relaxed and didn't do my one day of maintenance each week I immediately felt the weight going back on, so now I know that to keep the weight off this needs to be a way of life. But because it's only one day I find it easy to do – everyone can be "good" one day a week! It doesn't really impact on my lifestyle and I can adjust it to suit times like holidays and Christmas. The one time when I struggle is when I am unhappy – then I still crave comfort food. I suppose the answer is to be happy all the time!'

8. Get peer support from other maintainers

It can be enormously helpful to have regular contact with other people who are also trying to keep the weight off. To help you keep on track with your weight maintenance, as well as your dieting, visit our website www.thetwodaydiet.co.uk or find us on Facebook, where you can get support and ideas from other maintainers.

What happens if my weight creeps back up again?

If you start to notice your weight is increasing, keep a close eye on it. Weight can vary from day to day by as much as 2–4 lb (1–1.8 kg), but if you notice a gradual increase over three or four weeks, then you need to take action straight away. It's relatively easy to shed a few extra pounds, but when that turns into half a stone (3 kg) it becomes much more difficult. If the weight gain is literally just a pound or two (0.5–1 kg) and you want to get rid of it, check and adjust your diet over the next few weeks and increase your exercise. If you have regained more than this, you should go back onto The 2-Day Diet for a few weeks until you have lost the regained weight – and then go immediately back to The 1-Day Maintenance Diet.

Have you reached your goal or are you stuck?

If you have achieved the weight you were aiming for or are happy with the amount that you have lost, then follow The 1-Day Maintenance Diet. However, if you feel that you are stuck at a particular weight and unable to move on and you're reading this chapter because you feel like giving up on your weight-loss goal, whatever you do – don't! Although we expect your rate of weight loss to gradually decrease over six to eight months, it shouldn't grind to a halt. In fact, several studies of Dieters under controlled conditions have found that although the majority of weight loss does happen in the first six to eight months, your weight should continue to gradually drop over three years – and then it will reach a plateau. So you would lose half of the total weight you lose in the first year and the second half in the following two years[3].

If your weight loss has ground to a halt, then it's time to go back to basics. The reduction in your metabolic rate could be an important factor in slowing down your weight loss, but it shouldn't stop it altogether. The main reason why weight loss reaches a plateau is because, understandably, people become less vigilant about their diet and exercise regime over time without even realising it's happening. It may be a few weeks since you stopped being as rigorous about your diet and exercise as you were, but assumed it was okay because you kept losing weight until you eventually plateau-ed. Check that you really are sticking to eating and exercise plans as carefully as you were in week one of your 2-Day Diet. If you are not following these plans to the letter, as you were when you started the Diet, go back to those chapters (see pages 44 and 117) and remind yourself of the rules. To get back on track, it may help to keep a diet and exercise diary to record your eating and activity levels.

CASE STUDY: Linda

Linda, 31, started to gain weight in her mid 20s and was 11 stone 4 lb (71.6 kg) by the time she started The 2-Day Diet. 'I had always been active and a healthy weight, but a combination of university and a love for triple chocolate muffins meant that I went from a size 10 to a size 14 and my weight shot up from 9 stone 11 lb (62 kg) to a not-so-healthy 12 stone (76 kg). I lost a bit of weight over the next few years, but I was still around 10 stone 10 lb (68 kg) and although I had a relatively healthy diet, my serving sizes were way out of control and I did no exercise. After one Christmas when my weight had gone up to 11 stone 3 lb (71.2 kg) and my mum had developed severe complications of diabetes I realised that I had to do something about my weight or I would make myself ill.

I'd started exercising more, but it usually left me really hungry and my weight loss was slow, probably because I was overeating. I decided on The 2-Day Diet because I don't have the will power for seven days a week. I'm vegetarian so the low-carb days made me look carefully at what I was eating and see where there were imbalances.

With the added incentive of my wedding, I decided that 2012 was a sink-or-swim year. The diet was quite hard at first and I was hungry by Day Two, but the two days left me feeling lighter and somehow 'cleaner' on the inside. A few weeks into it, I didn't notice the hunger any more, but the thing I really liked was that I could choose which two consecutive days to do. So if we had planned a meal out, I'd switch my days so I wasn't restricting myself that day. Crucially, I didn't feel as though I was missing out. Only restricting myself for two days also meant that I had the energy to exercise on the other days – something I don't think I could have stuck at if the restriction had been continuous.

My weight loss has been gradual, but maintained. You have to spend the first couple of weeks getting used to the Diet, but the longer you stick with it – the easier it gets. And I finally understand serving sizes. Best of all I was a size 10 for my wedding!'

Summary

▶ Congratulate yourself on your weight-loss success! You have achieved the weight you were aiming for and are likely to have permanently improved your health and retrained your eating habits.

▶ Because you now weigh less, your body needs fewer calories to function. The tried-and-tested 1-Day Maintenance Diet is designed to ensure that you keep the weight off.

▶ The 1-Day Maintenance Diet involves doing one restricted day every week, six days of an unrestricted Mediterranean diet and maintaining your activity levels (300 minutes per week). This should enable you to keep your new weight stable.

▶ Key elements of successful maintenance are regular monitoring of your weight and serving sizes, staying active, setting a new goal and reward system for yourself, and getting the support you need.

▶ If your weight has plateau-ed and you would like to lose more, go back the basics of The 2-Day Diet (see page 44) and repeat your goal-setting and monitoring.

8

meal
planners

Here are some suggested meal plans to help guide you through
the early weeks of The 2-Day Diet – until the two-day pattern
of eating becomes established. We've given you four weeks of
menu suggestions with the restricted days falling on a Monday
and Tuesday, as many of our Dieters chose these two days as
their diet days. You can, of course, swap them around if other
days work better for you. It is probably a good idea to try as
much as possible to stick to the same two days each week so
The 2-day Diet becomes a habit. However, the beauty of the
Diet is that you can move the days to fit into your week.

This chapter includes both standard and vegetarian plans
that combine easy-to-prepare recipes with quick, healthy
meals. When you reach the end of Week Four you can go back
to the beginning, adding in some of the other recipes that
you'll find in chapters 9 and 10.

Use the planner in the way that works best for you. Some Dieters find that sticking closely to suggested meal plans helps them to keep focused, especially at the beginning of The 2-Day Diet. For those who want more flexibility, the meal plans will provide a great starting point to mix and match meal ideas. Drinks have not been included on these meal plans, but it is important to drink 2 litres (4 pints) per day. Two dairy portions have been included on each day and it is assumed that one additional dairy portion will be used as milk in drinks throughout the day.

The 2-Day Diet

Week 1

Meal	Monday	Tuesday	Wednesday	Thursday	Friday	Saturday	Sunday
Breakfast	Grilled bacon and plum tomatoes Milky coffee	Recipe: Eggs on a bed of spinach	Recipe: Porridge with dried fruit	Wheat or oat 'bisk' cereal with milk	Bran-based cereal and milk	Wholemeal toast, olive spread and low-sugar jam	Recipe: Classic muesli
Mid-morning snack							Handful of Brazil nuts
Lunch	Recipe: Cauliflower soup	Vegetable crudités with low-fat hummus and low-fat cream cheese	Recipe: Tuna and mixed bean salad Yoghurt	Recipe: Warm beetroot and feta salad, served with new potatoes	Recipe: Lentil soup with spinach and a touch of lemon, served with a chicken salad sandwich on wholemeal bread with low-fat mayonnaise	Wholewheat crackers with lowfat cream cheese plus mixed salad with salmon, butter beans, with olive oil dressing	Rye toast with low-fat spread and baked beans
Mid-afternoon snack	Slice of melon	Handful of pistachio nuts	Apple	Handful of mixed unsalted nuts		Apple	Glass of vegetable juice
Evening meal	Recipe: Stuffed mackerel served with large serving of steamed broccoli	Recipe: Chicken or turkey stir-fry with mangetout and green beans Strawberries and yoghurt	Recipe: Baked chicken with rosemary, served with bulgar wheat and three servings of steamed vegetables	Recipe: Beef meatballs with sauce and wholewheat spaghetti; served with large mixed salad Recipe: Prune delight	Grilled sardines served with new potatoes and two servings of steamed vegetables Recipe: Baked nectarines stuffed with nuts	Recipe: Chicken fajitas, served with large mixed salad Recipe: Yoghurt ice cream with raspberries	Recipe: Aubergine curry with chickpeas, rice and a mango raita
Supper	Handful of almonds		Olives		Vegetable crudités and tomato salsa		Clementine, small glass of milk

Week 2

Meal	Monday	Tuesday	Wednesday	Thursday	Friday	Saturday	Sunday
Breakfast	Half a grapefruit. Recipe: Spicy scrambled eggs	Recipe: Papaya and golden linseed smoothie	Bran flakes and milk	Granary toast with peanut butter	Wheat or oat 'bisk' cereal with milk	Kipper with wholemeal toast and spread	Recipe: Porridge with dried fruit
Mid-morning snack			Grapes		Fat-free fromage frais		Pear
Lunch	Recipe: Zingy smoked salmon salad with avocado	Recipe: Chinese vegetable soup with tofu	Recipe: Creamy mushroom soup, served with a ham and salad wholemeal bread roll with low-fat spread. Yoghurt	Recipe: White bean salad with hard-boiled eggs, served with wholemeal crackers and low-fat cream cheese	Granary toast with low-fat spread and a tin of sardines in tomato sauce. Glass of vegetable juice	Recipe: Horiatiki salata – Greek salad – served with granary bread	Recipe: Courgette soup with basil and tomato salsa, and a chicken and salad sandwich on a wholemeal roll
Mid-afternoon snack	Piece of Edam	Handful of Brazil nuts	Two satsumas		Small apple	Handful of mixed unsalted nuts	
Evening meal	Recipe: Tangy chicken drumsticks with crudités and a harissa dip	Recipe: White fish with tangy watercress sauce, served with two servings of steamed vegetables	Recipe: Prawns with beans, tomatoes and thyme, served with brown rice and mixed green salad	Olives. Recipe: Marinated lamb and red onion kebabs with a yoghurt and herb sauce, served with new potatoes and large mixed salad or three servings of vegetables. Recipe: Apricot and apple fruit salad	Recipe: Courgette frittata, served with baked potato and a large salad with mixed salad beans. Yoghurt ice cream with raspberries	Recipe: Chicken tagine with carrots and chickpeas, served with couscous. Fruit and yoghurt	Recipe: Roasted vegetables with grilled low-fat halloumi, served with homemade potato wedges and green salad
Supper	Handful of pistachio nuts	Cherry tomatoes	Handful of unsalted peanuts				Yoghurt

Week 3

Meal	Monday	Tuesday	Wednesday	Thursday	Friday	Saturday	Sunday
Breakfast	Recipe: Eggs on a bed of spinach	Grilled bacon and tomatoes with mushrooms fried in olive oil

Milky coffee | Branflakes with mixed seeds and milk | Scrambled egg and tinned plum tomatoes on rye toast

Glass of milk | Fruit and fibre cereal with milk | Granary toast and olive spread with mushrooms fried in olive oil, grilled tomatoes and a poached egg | Bran-based cereal with chopped, mixed nuts and milk |
| Mid-morning snack | | | | Pear | | Plums | Strawberries and yoghurt |
| Lunch | Recipe: Chicken soup

Handful of unsalted mixed nuts | Tuna salad made with tinned tuna and an olive oil dressing | Recipe: Roast red pepper soup, served with granary bread and low-fat hummus

Tangerines | Salmon and cucumber sandwiches made with tinned salmon and granary bread

Yoghurt | Recipe: Tabbouleh with low-fat hummus | Baked potato, baked beans and grated low-fat Cheddar | Recipe: A pair of potato salads (the smoked mackerel version) |
| Mid-afternoon snack | Summer berry smoothie made with frozen mixed berries, milk, yoghurt and vanilla essence | | Yoghurt | | Apple, handful of pistachio nuts | Glass of vegetable juice | Recipe: Guacamole, served with carrot sticks |
| Evening meal | Recipe: Lamb chops and 'little dishes' | Recipe: Quick cauliflower and okra curry with a yoghurt and mint raita

Strawberries | Recipe: Mediterranean chicken casserole served with three servings of steamed vegetables and bulgar wheat

Recipe: Chocolate and orange mousse | Recipe: Red pepper, courgette and mushroom lasagne, served with a side salad | Recipe: Bean and green pepper chilli with brown rice

Recipe: Blackberry and apple crumble, served with fat-free Greek yoghurt | Corn on the cob Recipe: Black peppered salmon steak, served with two servings of steamed vegetables

Recipe: Crunchy blackberry and apple crumble | Recipe: Thai-style stir-fried beef with lime, red onion and cucumber served with wholemeal boiled noodles |
| Supper | Piece of Bavarian smoked cheese | Handful of unsalted Brazil nuts | | Grapes | | | Dried apricots |

Week 4

Meal	Monday	Tuesday	Wednesday	Thursday	Friday	Saturday	Sunday
Breakfast	Grilled kipper with grilled tomatoes	Recipe: Greek yoghurt with blackberries and cinnamon-toasted cashews	Recipe: Porridge with dried fruit	Wheat or oat 'bisk' cereal with milk	Bran flakes and milk. Glass of pineapple juice	Granary toast and peanut butter	Recipe: Classic muesli
Mid-morning snack				Pear		Glass of milk	Apricot
Lunch	Recipe: Iced cucumber soup. Piece of low-fat Cheddar and piece of Bavarian smoked cheese	Ham and cottage cheese salad. Handful of walnuts	Grilled chicken breast salad (lettuce, cucumber and tomatoes) served with oatcakes and low-fat cream cheese	Recipe: Creamy mushroom soup, served with rye crispbreads and low-fat hummus. Banana	Recipe: Courgette soup with basil and a tomato salsa. Sliced egg and salad sandwich on granary bread	Baked potato with tuna and low-fat mayonnaise, served with a green salad	Baked beans with granary toast with grated low-fat Cheddar
Mid-afternoon snack	Handful of Pistachio nuts	Boiled egg and cherry tomatoes	Glass of vegetable juice			Recipe: tsatsiki, served with cucumber and red pepper crudités	Glass of vegetable juice
Evening meal	Recipe: Griddled turkey steaks with garlic spinach. Slice of melon	Recipe: Prawn and vegetable kebabs	Recipe: Salmon with lentils, served with two servings of steamed vegetables or a large mixed salad. Recipe: Crêpe with honey	Chilli made with lean mince with added red kidney beans, served with brown rice, a dollop of plain yoghurt, and a tomato and cucumber salad	Recipe: Baked chicken with rosemary, served with boiled potatoes in their skins and two servings of steamed vegetables. Fruit and fat-free fromage frais	Recipe: Aubergine curry with chickpeas, rice (or a wholemeal chapatti) and mango raita. Recipe: Baked nectarines stuffed with nuts	Recipe: Smoked fish cakes served with a mixed salad
Supper			2 satsumas	Handful of unsalted peanuts		Banana	

Week 1 (vegetarian)

Meal	Monday	Tuesday	Wednesday	Thursday	Friday	Saturday	Sunday
Breakfast	Poached eggs and plum tomatoes	Recipe: Eggs on a bed of spinach	Wheat or oat 'bisk' cereal with milk and dried fruit	Recipe: Porridge with dried fruit	Granary toast and olive spread with grilled vegetarian sausages, grilled tomatoes and mushrooms fried in olive oil. Glass of orange juice	Recipe: Classic muesli	Wholemeal toast, olive spread and low-sugar jam
Mid-morning snack	Tofu strips sautéed in spices		Handful of pistachios				
Lunch	Recipe: Cauliflower soup	Vegetable crudités with low-fat hummus and low-fat cream cheese	Recipe: Courgette soup with basil with oatcakes and hummus	Rye crispbreads with low-fat cream cheese plus mixed salad with salad beans and olive oil dressing	Recipe: Lentil soup with spinach and a touch of lemon, served with oatcakes or a slice of wholemeal bread and olive spread	Rye toast with lowfat spread and baked beans or Recipe: Boston baked beans	Boiled egg and butter bean pasta salad (lettuce, spring onions and tomatoes) with olive oil dressing
Mid-afternoon snack	Glass of milk	Handful of mixed unsalted nuts	Apple	Glass of vegetable juice	Yoghurt	Low-fat hummus with celery and cucumber crudités	
Evening meal	Recipe: Oriental vegetable stir-fry with marinated tofu and cashews. Stewed rhubarb with sweeteners added to taste, with fat-free Greek yoghurt	Recipe: Italian bean stew. Strawberries and yoghurt	Recipe: Pasta Arrabbiata with tofu, served with two servings of steamed vegetables. Yoghurt	Recipe: Homemade classic burgers (V alternative) with new potatoes and two servings of steamed vegetables. Recipe: Yoghurt ice cream with raspberries	Homemade pizza – use a wholemeal pizza base and a tomato purée, olive oil and garlic base with vegetables (onions, peppers, sweetcorn, mushrooms, olives) and mozzarella cheese on top. Serve with large salad	Recipe: Warm beetroot and feta salad, served with new potatoes and sliced egg. Satsuma	Recipe: Aubergine curry with chickpeas, rice and a mango raita. Recipe: Prune delight, served with yoghurt
Supper	Handful of unsalted peanuts	Boiled eggs	Olives		Peach	Handful of Brazil nuts	

Week 2 (vegetarian)

Meal	Monday	Tuesday	Wednesday	Thursday	Friday	Saturday	Sunday
Breakfast	Half a grapefruit / Recipe: Spicy scrambled eggs	Recipe: Papaya and golden linseed smoothie	Bran flakes and milk	Granary toast with peanut butter	Wheat or oat 'bisk' cereal with milk / Glass of fruit juice	Wholemeal toast and poached egg	Recipe: Porridge with dried fruit and honey
Mid-morning snack	Piece of Edam	Boiled egg			Fat-free fromage frais		Plum
Lunch	Recipe: Mint, feta and soya bean salad	Recipe: Chinese vegetable soup with tofu	Recipe: Creamy mushroom soup, served with wholemeal crackers and low-fat hummus / Handful of unsalted peanuts	Recipe: White bean salad with hardboiled eggs, served with oatcakes and low-fat soft white cheese	Recipe: Courgette soup with basil and a tomato salsa, served with oatcakes and low-fat hummus	Recipe: Horiatiki salata (Greek salad), served with granary bread	Recipe: Boston beans, served with baked potato
Mid-afternoon snack	Handful of Brazil nuts		Pear	Cherry tomatoes	Banana		Low-fat cream cheese with carrot and cucumber sticks
Evening meal	Recipe: Ginger, soy and chilli tofu skewers with Chinese leaf and mangetout salad	Recipe: Cauliflower and mushroom curry with yoghurt (add tofu if you want extra bulk)	Recipe: Bean and green pepper chilli served with a green salad / Fruit and yoghurt	Olives / Recipe: Crunchy stuffed pepper with rocket and raita, served with (Recipe) Red cabbage coleslaw with nuts and seeds / Recipe: Apricot and apple fruit salad	Bean and vegetable bake (Adapted Recipe: Prawns with beans, tomatoes and thyme – make this without prawns and instead soften onions and peppers in the oil before adding the tomatoes, and serve with a mashed potato topping)	Recipe: Courgette frittata, served with baked potato and salad with mixed salad beans / Recipe: Blackberry and apple crumble, served with fromage frais	Recipe: Orzotto with peas and broad beans
Supper		Handful of mixed unsalted nuts		Glass of milk			Handful of walnuts

Week 3 (vegetarian)

Meal	Monday	Tuesday	Wednesday	Thursday	Friday	Saturday	Sunday
Breakfast	Recipe: Greek yoghurt with blackberries and cinamon-toasted cashews	Recipe: Eggs on a bed of spinach	Fruit and fibre cereal and milk	Scrambled egg and tinned plum tomatoes on rye toast; Glass of milk	Granary toast with olive spread, with mushrooms fried in olive oil, grilled tomatoes and a poached egg	Bran flakes with mixed seeds and milk	Muesli and milk
Mid-morning snack						Banana smoothie made with semiskimmed milk and natural yoghurt	
Lunch	Recipe: Cauliflower soup; Tofu strips stir fried in spices with sesame seeds	Mozzarella and tomato salad served with green salad and olive oil dressing	Vegetarian sausage sandwich on a wholemeal roll, with a large side salad	Recipe: A pair of potato salads (the vegetarian version); Mixed pepper sticks and lowfat hummus	Recipe: Roast red pepper soup, served with rye crispbreads and low-fat hummus	Recipe: White bean salad with hard-boiled eggs, served with a slice of wholemeal bread and low-fat spread	Low-fat hummus and grated carrot sandwiches on granary bread, with side salad; Strawberries and yoghurt
Mid-afternoon snack	Handful of almonds	Glass of vegetable juice		Kiwi fruit		Apple	Handful of unsalted mixed nuts
Evening meal	Recipe: Fluffy omelette with spring onions and cheese served with a large mixed salad	Recipe: Oriental vegetable stir-fry with marinated tofu and cashews; Slice of melon	Recipe: Bean and green pepper chilli with wholemeal basmati rice or a wholemeal chapatti and low fat plain yoghurt to serve; Recipe: Apricot and apple fruit salad	Recipe: Pasta Arrabiata with tofu, served with a side salad; Banana and yoghurt	Corn on the cob; Recipe: Roasted vegetables with grilled halloumi; Recipe: Crunchy blackberry and apple crumble and 1 portion custard (sweeten to taste with sweeteners)	Recipe: Red pepper, courgette and mushroom lasagne, served with a large salad	Recipe: Baked eggs Tunisian style; Recipe: Chocolate and orange mousse
Supper	Cottage cheese and crudités	Low-fat hummus and crudités					Plum

Week 4 (vegetarian)

Meal	Monday	Tuesday	Wednesday	Thursday	Friday	Saturday	Sunday
Breakfast	Grilled vegetarian sausages and tomatoes	Recipe: Spicy scrambled eggs	Recipe: Porridge with dried fruit	Wheat or oat 'bisk' cereal with milk	Grilled vegetarian sausage sandwich on a granary roll with grilled tomatoes Glass of milk	Fruit and fibre cereal and milk Glass of pineapple juice	Tomato omelette with wholemeal toast and lowfat spread
Mid-morning snack	Boiled egg	Apricots		Orange		Recipe: Guacamole served with crudités	
Lunch	Recipe: Iced cucumber soup Spiced stir-fried tofu strips	Recipe: Mint, feta and soya bean salad	Baked beans on granary toast	Sliced egg and salad sandwich on granary bread, served with (Recipe) Red cabbage coleslaw with nuts and seeds	Oatcakes served with olives, low-fat hummus and vegetable crudités	Poached egg and granary toast soldiers	Recipe: Creamy mushroom soup, served with rye crispbreads with low-fat cream cheese and cucumber
Mid-afternoon snack	Handful of pistachio nuts	Handful of Brazil nuts	Cherry tomatoes	Banana		Slice of melon	Pear
Evening meal	Recipe: Stuffed Portobello mushrooms Slice of melon	Recipe: Ginger, soy and chilli skewers with Chinese leaf and mange tout salad	Recipe: Crunchy stuffed peppers with rocket and raita, served with tomato salsa Fruit and yoghurt	Recipe: Courgette frittata with steamed vegetables Recipe: Lemon and honey cheesecake	Recipe: Bean and green pepper chilli, served with brown rice Recipe: Baked nectarines stuffed with nuts, served with yoghurt	Recipe: Roasted vegetables with halloumi, served with quinoa Recipe: Crêpes with honey	Adapted recipe: Italian bean stew with TVP added to the tomatoes and a mashed potato topping served with steamed vegetables Recipe: Lemon and blueberry yoghurt cake
Supper		Cottage cheese and cucumber sticks		Glass of vegetable juice			

9

recipes for the two restricted days

General note

Most recipes serve one to two people. If you are increasing quantities to feed more people, bear in mind that you may also need to adjust the cooking time. In some cases making a single portion is impractical – curries, soups and stews, espe- cially – and any excess can always be frozen, so that you have a stock of healthy ready meals.

All spoon measurements are level unless otherwise indicated and are assumed to be standard sizes: teaspoon = 5 ml; tablespoon = 15 ml. If you are in any doubt, get a set of spoon measures.

All hobs and ovens differ, so do check as you cook. The oven temperatures given are for conventional electric ovens and gas ovens; for fan-assisted ovens, subtract 20°C from the suggested cooking time.

Salt and sugar

Many of us have developed a preference for salty and sugary foods due to years of eating salty and sweet manufactured foods or habitually adding salt and sugar to flavour our food. Reducing salt and sugar intake is an important component of healthy eating. Cutting down on salt and sugar is quite straightforward: you simply need to get used to eating less.

Initially, when you reduce your salt and sugar intake, foods may taste bland or different. You can cut down on salt straight away or reduce your salt intake in 20 per cent steps. Most people can't taste the difference if they reduce salt gradually. Either way, after two or three weeks you will start to taste the genuine, delicious flavours of food. The recipes below include lots of alternative flavourings and do not require salt. Some recipes contain stock and we suggest that you use no more than 2 g/¼ stock cube per serving. You can use less than this if you wish or a low-salt bouillon. Try to use tuna, beans and pulses that are tinned in water and not brine or salted water. Similarly, try to use raw prawns, rather than cooked, as these contain much less salt: 100 g (3½ oz) of cooked prawns typically contain 1.1–2 g salt whereas raw prawns contain 0.5 g.

Recipes for your two restricted days

Breakfast	Page
Greek yoghurt with blackberries and cinnamon-toasted cashews (V)	184
Spicy scrambled eggs (V)	184
Smoked salmon and spinach wraps with cottage cheese and lemon	185
Eggs on a bed of spinach (V)	186
Papaya and golden linseed smoothie (V)	187
Soups	
Hot and sour prawn soup	187
Chinese vegetable soup with tofu (V)	188

Each recipe shows how many servings it contributes to your allowance in The 2-Day Diet plan. Many foods contain a combination of nutrients, some of which are in such small quantities they do not count towards your serving allowances. All servings have been rounded to the nearest half.

Breakfast

Greek yoghurt with blackberries and cinnamon-toasted cashews
Serves 1

10 unsalted cashew nuts
  pinch of ground
  cinnamon
80 g (2¾ oz) blackberries
120 g (4 oz) low-fat Greek
  yoghurt

SERVINGS		NUTRITIONAL INFO	
Protein	0	Calories	172
Fat	1	Carbohydrate	15 g
Dairy	1	Protein	9 g
Fruit	1	Fibre	5 g
Vegetables	0	Salt	0.3 g

Place a small frying pan over a medium heat. When hot, add the cashews and cinnamon to the pan and toast for 1–2 minutes, stirring occasionally with a wooden spoon, until golden and aromatic. Remove onto a chopping board and when cool enough to handle, roughly chop the nuts.

Spoon the yoghurt into a bowl and top with the blackberries. Finish by sprinkling over the cinnamon cashews.

Spicy scrambled eggs
Serves 1

2 eggs
½ tsp rapeseed oil
3 spring onions, chopped
½ mild chilli or to taste,
  finely chopped (optional)
¼ tsp turmeric
handful of coriander leaves

SERVINGS		NUTRITIONAL INFO	
Protein	2	Calories	228
Fat	0	Carbohydrate	4 g
Dairy	0	Protein	17 g
Fruit	0	Fibre	2 g
Vegetables	1½	Salt	0.5 g

1 medium tomato, chopped

Beat the eggs in a mug or bowl with a tablespoon of water.

Put the oil in a small non-stick pan over a medium heat. When hot, add the spring onions and chilli (if using) to the pan, and cook gently until the spring onions just begin to colour.

Add the turmeric and coriander leaves to the pan and stir for a few seconds, then add the tomato and continue stirring until the tomato is warmed through. Finally, add the beaten egg and cook, stirring constantly, until the egg begins to set. Remove the pan from the heat and serve immediately.

Smoked salmon and spinach wraps with cottage cheese and lemon

Serves 1

60 g (2 oz) smoked salmon slices
80 g (2¾ oz) baby spinach, washed and thoroughly dried
75 g (2½ oz) cottage cheese
zest of half a lemon
black pepper, to serve

SERVINGS		NUTRITIONAL INFO	
Protein	2	Calories	181
Fat	0	Carbohydrate	4 g
Dairy	1	Protein	27 g
Fruit	0	Fibre	2 g
Vegetables	1	Salt	3.7 g

Lay the slices of smoked salmon out onto a chopping board and sprinkle over the spinach leaves, making sure to contain them within the edges of the salmon slices. Spoon some cottage cheese along the centre of each slice and season with the lemon zest and a grind of black pepper. Roll up each salmon slice and serve immediately.

Eggs on a bed of spinach

Serves 1

100 g (3½ oz) baby spinach leaves
black pepper
dash of vinegar
2 eggs

SERVINGS		NUTRITIONAL INFO	
Protein	2	Calories	210
Fat	0	Carbohydrate	2 g
Dairy	0	Protein	18 g
Fruit	0	Fibre	3 g
Vegetables	1	Salt	0.8 g

Wash the spinach leaves and chop them roughly. Put the leaves into a pan over a medium heat, add a couple of twists of black pepper, cover and cook until the spinach begins to wilt. The water clinging to the leaves after washing will provide enough moisture to cook the spinach. Only cook the leaves until they have wilted down.

Fill a small pan with about 2 cm (½ in) water and add a little vinegar. Bring the water to the boil. Crack each egg into a cup or small jug. When the water is boiling, slide the eggs into the pan and reduce the heat to a simmer (if you are using an electric hob, you can switch the ring off). Cover the pan and allow the eggs to poach until they are done to your taste – 3 minutes or so should produce a set white and a runny yolk.

Drain the spinach well and put it on a warmed plate; spread it out. Lift the eggs from the pan with a slotted spoon so that the water drains away, and place them on top of the spinach. Add a little pepper to taste and serve immediately.

Papaya and golden linseed smoothie
Serves 1

120 g (4 oz) low-fat natural
    yoghurt
juice of half a lime
80 g (2¾ oz) ripe papaya,
    skinned and deseeded
1 tsp golden linseeds
5 ice cubes

SERVINGS		NUTRITIONAL INFO	
Protein	0	Calories	112
Fat	½	Carbohydrate	14 g
Dairy	1	Protein	7 g
Fruit	1	Fibre	3 g
Vegetables	0	Salt	0.2 g

Pour the yoghurt and lime juice into a blender and add the papaya. Blend until smooth (alternatively use a stick blender) and pour into a large glass over ice. Sprinkle over the linseeds and serve immediately.

Soups

Hot and sour prawn soup
Serves 1

350 ml (12 fl oz) low-salt fish
    or vegetable stock
½ tsp fish sauce (optional)
1 small red chilli, finely chopped
juice of half a lime
½ tsp low-salt soy sauce
2 cm (½ in) piece of ginger,
    finely grated
1 stick lemongrass, outer leaves
    removed, finely sliced
180 g (6 oz) raw tiger prawns

SERVINGS		NUTRITIONAL INFO	
Protein	4	Calories	175
Fat	0	Carbohydrate	5 g
Dairy	0	Protein	35 g
Fruit	0	Fibre	2 g
Vegetables	1	Salt	2.1 g

1 spring onion, finely sliced
3 cherry tomatoes, halved
7 button mushrooms, halve
1 tbsp chopped coriander

Pour the hot fish stock into a saucepan and add the fish sauce, chilli, lime juice, soy sauce, ginger and lemongrass and place over a medium heat. Bring to a boil, lower the heat and simmer for 3–4 minutes, until fragrant. Add the prawns, spring onion, tomatoes and mushrooms and simmer for a further 2 minutes, until the prawns have turned pink. Serve immediately, sprinkled with the coriander.

Chinese vegetable soup with tofu
Serves 1

250 ml (8½ fl oz) low-salt vegetable stock
1 small pak choi or half a large one, trimmed (about 60 g/2 oz)
3 button mushrooms, finely sliced
3 spring onions, trimmed and finely sliced
1 small piece fresh ginger root (about 6 g)

1 garlic clove
150 g (5 oz) firm tofu
dash of light soy sauce

SERVINGS		NUTRITIONAL INFO	
Protein	3	Calories	149
Fat	0	Carbohydrate	6 g
Dairy	0	Protein	15 g
Fruit	0	Fibre	4 g
Vegetables	1½	Salt	1.2 g

Put the stock in a pan and bring it to the boil. Separate the pak choi leaves then slice the stems into thin sticks and the leaves into strips. Put the stems into the stock, together with the mushrooms and the spring onions and lower the heat to a simmer. Grate the ginger and garlic into the pan and cook for 3 minutes.

Cut the tofu into pieces about 1.5 cm (½ in) square. Add the sliced pak choi leaves to the pan and stir them in.

Then gently put the tofu in the pan and simmer for a further 2 minutes.

Take the pan off the heat, then using a slotted spoon lift the vegetables and tofu into a serving bowl. Carefully pour the liquid on top and serve immediately with a dash of light soy sauce.

Tip:

▶ Not suitable for freezing.

Cauliflower soup

Serves 1, generously

1 small cauliflower
 (about 200 g/7 oz)
½ tsp rapeseed oil
½ leek, chopped
 (about 80 g/2¾ oz)
1 garlic clove, crushed
500 ml (17½ fl oz) low-salt
 vegetable stock
100–150 ml (3½–5 fl oz)
 semi-skimmed or
 skimmed milk
black pepper

SERVINGS		NUTRITIONAL INFO	
using semi- skimmed milk			
Protein	0	Calorie	182
Fat	0	Carbohydrate	17 g
Dairy	½	Protein	14 g
Fruit	0	Fibre	7 g
Vegetables	3½	Salt	1.1 g

Trim the outer leaves from the cauliflower and split it into florets, cutting away the central stalk – there should be 175 g (6 oz) of cauliflower remaining.

Heat the oil in a pan and add the leek. Stir it for a minute, then add the cauliflower florets and the garlic. Stir these around for a further minute, but don't let them brown; then add the stock. Bring the stock to the boil, reduce the heat and simmer uncovered, until the cauliflower and leek are soft and the liquid is much reduced – about 15 minutes.

Remove the pan from the heat. Blend the soup using a hand blender or place the contents in a liquidiser and blitz, adding enough milk to reach a consistency you like. Return the soup to the pan (if you've used a blender), add black pepper to taste, then reheat and serve.

Tip:

▶ This simple and delicious soup is suitable for making in batches and freezing – just multiply the ingredients as required.

Chicken soup
Serves 1

*1 chicken breast, skin
    removed, about 150 g
    (5 oz)
500 ml (17½ fl oz) low-salt
    vegetable stock
1 small bay leaf
sprig of thyme
1 leek, trimmed
    (about 160 g/5½ oz)
3 green or runner beans, cut
    into 2 cm (½ in) lengths*

SERVINGS		NUTRITIONAL INFO	
Protein	5	Calories	239
Fat	0	Carbohydrate	9 g
Dairy	0	Protein	39 g
Fruit	0	Fibre	6 g
Vegetables	3	Salt	1.2 g

*50 ml (1¾ fl oz) semi-
    skimmed milk (optional)*

Put the whole chicken breast into a pan with the stock. Add the bay leaf and thyme sprig, bring the stock to the boil, then reduce the heat and simmer for 10 minutes.

Divide the leek into green and white parts, then chop the green part and add it to the pan. Simmer for a further 10 minutes. While simmering chop the rest of the leek and add to the stock with the beans.

Continue simmering for 5 more minutes, by which time the chicken should be tender and cooked through; cook a little longer if necessary.

Carefully lift the chicken out of the pan with a slotted spoon and chop it into cubes no larger than 2 cm (½ in). Remove the bay leaf and the woody stem of the thyme sprig from the stock. Return the chicken pieces to the pan and increase the temperature to reduce the liquid and reheat the chicken. This will take about 5 minutes.

To serve you can either:

▶ Eat the soup as it is with small cubes of chicken and vegetables in a beautifully flavoured broth.

▶ Ladle the liquid and some of the vegetables into a jug, add the milk, blitz together with a hand-held blender, then return the liquid to the pan.

▶ Add the milk to the pan and blend everything together into a smooth soup using a hand-held blender (or blitz using a liquidiser and return to the pan).

Whatever you decide, reheat the soup and season with black pepper before serving.

Tips:

▶ You could substitute the beans for another green vegetable (see page 53).

▶ This soup is suitable for making in batches and freezing – simply multiply the ingredients as required.

Iced cucumber soup

Serves 1

½ small cucumber, peeled
   and chopped
½ leek, trimmed and chopped
½ tsp rapeseed oil
150 ml (5 fl oz) semi-
   skimmed milk
½ tsp cornflour
150 ml (5 fl oz) low-salt
   vegetable stock
a few fresh chives, chopped
black pepper

SERVINGS		NUTRITIONAL INFO	
Protein	0	Calories	138
Fat	0	Carbohydrate	17 g
Dairy	1	Protein	7 g
Fruit	0	Fibre	3 g
Vegetables	3	Salt	0.7 g

Prepare the cucumber and leek, then heat the oil in a pan over a medium heat and add the chopped vegetables. Put the milk in a separate pan and warm it up.

Cover the pan with the cucumber and leeks and cook gently for about 5 minutes – check to make sure there is no sign of burning. Put the cornflour in a small bowl and add a little of the hot milk. Blend together until you have a smooth paste and then add it to the pan of vegetables. Stir well for a minute or so and then take the pan off the heat.

Gradually stir in the rest of the hot milk and the stock. Return the pan to the heat and bring it to the boil, then reduce the heat and simmer gently for 20 minutes. Blend the soup thoroughly and transfer it to a bowl when it is completely smooth (it should have the consistency of single cream). Allow the soup to cool, then cover the bowl and chill the soup in the refrigerator until completely cold.

When you are ready to serve, take the bowl out of the refrigerator and scatter some chopped chives over the surface. Add a little black pepper and serve immediately.

Tip:

▶ This soup needs to be eaten fresh and is not suitable for freezing. The cornflower provides 1 g of carbohydrate.

Japanese miso soup with shiitake mushrooms and greens

Serves 1

½ tbsp good-quality miso paste

300 ml (10 fl oz) freshly boiled water

½ tsp soy sauce

1 cm (¼ in) piece of root ginger, finely grated

2 spring onions, finely sliced

40 g (1½ oz) green spinach, washed

3 asparagus spears, sliced into 2 cm (½ in) pieces

3 shiitake mushrooms, sliced

¼ tsp toasted sesame seeds

SERVINGS		NUTRITIONAL INFO	
Protein	0	Calories	59
Fat	0	Carbohydrate	5 g
Dairy	0	Protein	5 g
Fruit	0	Fibre	4 g
Vegetables	1½	Salt	1.2 g

Put the miso paste in a small bowl and add 2–3 tablespoons of the boiling water to make a paste. Spoon the paste into a small saucepan and gradually stir in the remaining water to make a smooth stock. Add the soy sauce and ginger and bring to the boil. Lower the heat and simmer for 2–3 minutes before adding the spring onions, spinach, asparagus and mushrooms. Simmer for 2 minutes, add the sesame seeds and serve immediately.

Salads and light bites

Dips
Tsatsiki
Serves 1

*150 g (5 oz) low- or no-fat
    Greek yoghurt
1 small garlic clove, crushed
5 cm (2 in) piece of
    cucumber
large handful of coriander
    leaves
half a handful of mint leaves
    black pepper*

SERVINGS		NUTRITIONAL INFO	
Protein	0	Calories	103
Fat	0	Carbohydrate	15 g
Dairy	1	Protein	10 g
Fruit	0	Fibre	1 g
Vegetables	1	Salt	0.3 g

Put the yoghurt and crushed garlic into a bowl. Slice the cucumber in half and remove the seeds with a spoon, then finely chop the flesh. Add this to the yoghurt mixture.

Chop the coriander and mint leaves together and add them to the yoghurt, then stir everything together. Grind over some black pepper and serve immediately.

Guacamole
Serves 1

½ ripe avocado
squeeze lemon juice
1 spring onion, chopped
4 cherry tomatoes, chopped
½ small red chilli (or to taste), finely chopped

SERVINGS		NUTRITIONAL INFO	
Protein	0	Calories	155
Fat	2	Carbohydrate	4 g
Dairy	0	Protein	2 g
Fruit	0	Fibre	5 g
Vegetables	½	Salt	< 0.1 g

Remove the stone from the avocado. Slice through the flesh just to the skin lengthways, and then do the same across. Then bend the avocado back on itself – the flesh will either come out or will be very easy to remove, depending on its ripeness.

Put it in a bowl, add a little lemon juice and mash the flesh with a fork until there are no large pieces. Stir in the spring onion, tomatoes and chilli, check for seasoning and serve immediately.

Tip:
▶ Both these dips are great served with vegetable crudités or with iceberg lettuce leaves used as scoops.

Crab salad
Serves 1

1 x 170 g (6 oz) tin white crab meat or 100 g (3½ oz) fresh crab meat
2 tsp low-fat mayonnaise
zest and juice ½ unwaxed lemon

SERVINGS		NUTRITIONAL INFO	
Protein	4	Calories	316
Fat	2½	Carbohydrate	4 g
Dairy	0	Protein	22 g
Fruit	0	Fibre	5 g
Vegetables	1	Salt	1.4 g

few drops Tabasco sauce
  (optional)
black pepper
3 spring onions, trimmed

and chopped
½ avocado, stone removed
handful salad leaves
  (about 60 g/2 oz)

Drain the tin of crab into a sieve, rinse under running water and then set the sieve over a bowl to drain thoroughly. Omit this step if you are using fresh crab, but check the crab meat for any small pieces of shell.

Break up any chunks of crab meat very gently, using a fork and set aside.

Put the mayonnaise into a bowl and squeeze over a scant teaspoon of the lemon juice, then add the lemon zest to the mixture. Add the Tabasco, if using, and plenty of black pepper. Add the spring onions and stir everything together.

Slice lengthways through the flesh of the avocado just to the skin, and do the same across; then bend the avocado back on itself and remove the cubes of flesh. Put these in the bowl of mayonnaise and add the crab meat. Turn all the ingredients together gently, but make sure everything is incorporated.

Put some salad leaves on a plate and spoon the crab salad on top. Serve immediately.

Tuna pâté with crudités
Serves 1

1 x 160–185 g (5½–6½ oz) tin
  tuna steak in spring water
1 heaped tbsp low-fat cream
  cheese
1 heaped tbsp low- or no-fat

Greek yoghurt
squeeze or two of lemon juice
drop or two of Tabasco or
  Worcester sauce, to taste
black pepper

For the crudités:

3 celery sticks, trimmed and
cut into smaller sticks

6 spring onions, trimmed

5 cm (2 in) piece of
cucumber, cut into strips

SERVINGS		NUTRITIONAL INFO	
Protein	3½–4	Calories	228
Fat	0	Carbohydrate	7 g
Dairy	1½	Protein	35 g
Fruit	0	Fibre	4 g
Vegetables	3	Salt	0.6 g

Drain the tin of tuna. If you could only buy fish in brine, put it in a sieve and rinse under running water to remove excess salt.

Transfer the tuna to a bowl and break it up with a fork, then add the cream cheese and the yoghurt and mix together. Add a squeeze or two of lemon juice and, tasting carefully, a little Tabasco or Worcestershire sauce. Then add some black pepper and mix everything once more.

Cover the bowl and put the pâté in the refrigerator for at least 2 hours to allow the flavours to develop. Prepare the crudités just before serving.

Tips:

▶ This is a very adaptable recipe: for a firmer, more set pâté, use 2 tins of tuna; for a softer dip, use more yoghurt. Either way it is ideal for a packed lunch.

Zingy smoked salmon salad with avocado

Serves 1

75 g (2½ oz) smoked salmon
black pepper
1 lemon
2 cm (½ in) piece of
cucumber

1 tsp olive oil
½ tsp sesame seeds
small bunch watercress
small bunch rocket leaves
½ small avocado

Cut the smoked salmon into strips and put them in a bowl. Grind some black pepper over them and squeeze a little lemon juice over them as well; stir together. Cut the cucumber in half lengthways and

SERVINGS		NUTRITIONAL INFO	
Protein	2	Calories	226
Fat	2½	Carbohydrate	2 g
Dairy	0	Protein	22 g
Fruit	0	Fibre	3 g
Vegetables	1	Salt	3.6 g

remove the seeds, then cut each half in half again lengthways, and finely slice the cucumber sections. Add them to the smoked salmon. Set the bowl aside while you prepare the dressing and assemble the salad.

Put the olive oil in a small bowl and add a squeeze of lemon juice. Whisk or stir them together well and then scatter in the sesame seeds. Tear the leaves from the watercress stalks and put them on a serving plate with the rocket. Peel the avocado and cut it into fine slices. Put these around the salad, then spoon the salmon and cucumber mixture on top. Whisk up the dressing once more and drizzle it over the salad. Serve immediately.

Tip:

▶ As an alternative make this salad using fresh horseradish instead of the sesame seeds – when it is in season. Grate a little fresh root into the dressing about 30 minutes before assembling the salad. Fresh horseradish can be found at farmers' markets, in good greengrocers or online – and it's best in autumn and winter.

Fish and seafood

Chilli and pesto sea bream
Serves 1

2 sea bream fillets (weighing
about 120 g/4 oz each)
½ red chilli, finely chopped
1 tsp green pesto
juice and zest of ½ a lemon
a small handful of torn basil
leaves, to serve

SERVINGS		NUTRITIONAL INFO	
Protein	4	Calories	254
Fat	1	Carbohydrate	3 g
Dairy	0	Protein	36 g
Fruit	0	Fibre	3 g
Vegetables	1	Salt	0.9 g

For the kale:
100 g curly kale, tough central stalk cut out and leaves
shredded

Preheat grill to high.

Make 2 diagonal slices on the skin of each fillet and place on a lipped baking tray. Mix together the chilli, pesto, half the lemon juice and zest to make a marinade and pour over the fish – making sure that it is completely smothered on both sides. Set aside for 20 minutes.

Meanwhile, sprinkle the remaining lemon juice and zest over the kale and massage between your fingers to soften the pieces of kale, until it is slightly wilted. Set aside.

Grill the fish for 3 minutes each side until cooked through and the skin is crisp and slightly charred. Serve immediately on a bed of the kale and scatter the basil leaves on top.

Salmon parcels with aromatic salad
Serves 2

4 lemon slices

1 small onion, sliced into
   rings (for flavour only)

1 fennel bulb

2 salmon fillets, about 120 g
   (4 oz) each

1 bay leaf

sprig of thyme

2 handfuls of salad leaves

6 spring onions, finely sliced

10 cm (4 in) piece of
   cucumber, finely sliced

2 tsp olive oil (not extra
   virgin)

squeeze of lemon juice

black pepper

SERVINGS		NUTRITIONAL INFO	
Protein	4	Calories	276
Fat	½	Carbohydrate	4 g
Dairy	0	Protein	27 g
Fruit	0	Fibre	4 g
Vegetables	2	Salt	0.2 g

Preheat the oven to 200°C/400°F/Gas Mark 6.

Take a large piece of foil and put two lemon slices in the middle of it. Scatter the onion rings over the centre of the foil as well. Cut a vertical slice off the fennel bulb and add that too. Put the two salmon fillets on top and tuck the bay leaf and thyme sprig between them. Top each fillet with the remaining slices of lemon and bring the edges of the foil up around the fish and over the top. Fold the edges together to make a loose but well-sealed parcel.

Put the parcel in an ovenproof dish or roasting tin and cook for 15 minutes in the preheated oven. Remove the dish from the oven and carefully open the foil – the salmon should be almost cooked. Fold back the edges of the foil, exposing the fish, and remove the top two slices of lemon. Then put the dish back in the oven for a further 5 minutes or until the fish is cooked and opaque all the way through.

Remove the bay leaf and thyme, and carefully lift the salmon off the lemon, onion and fennel (discard these, along with the salmon skin).

Set the fish aside to cool slightly, and prepare the salad. Finely slice the rest of the fennel bulb, and combine with the salad leaves, spring onions and cucumber. Drizzle the olive oil over the salad, squeeze on the lemon juice and grind over some black pepper, then toss all the salad ingredients together. Serve immediately with the salmon.

Tip:

▶ This salmon is very good cold, perhaps served with the 'Almost a Celeri Remoulade' (see page 237) as an accompaniment instead of the fennel salad.

▶ Or try it with some lemon mayonnaise – put 1 tablespoon of low-fat mayonnaise in a small dish, grate over a little unwaxed lemon zest and mix well.

▶ For unrestricted days, serve with boiled new potatoes.

Grilled cod with spinach and asparagus served with quick-pickled radishes and cucumber

Serves 1

*1 skinless cod fillet, weighing
    about 120–180 g (4–6 oz)*
juice of half a lemon
black pepper
*2.5 cm (1 in) piece of
    cucumber, cut in half
    vertically and finely sliced*

SERVINGS		NUTRITIONAL INFO	
Protein	2–3	Calories	206
Fat	0	Carbohydrate	5 g
Dairy	0	Protein	39 g
Fruit	0	Fibre	5 g
Vegetables	2½	Salt	0.4 g

1 cm (¼ in) piece of ginger,
    very finely sliced
5 radishes, finely sliced
1½ tsp rice wine vinegar
¼ tsp toasted sesame seeds

40 g (1½ oz) baby leaf
    spinach
5 spears of asparagus, sliced
    into 5 cm (2 in) pieces

Preheat the oven to 180°C/350°F/Gas Mark 4.

Place the cod in a small ovenproof dish and sprinkle over the lemon juice. Season with black pepper and bake in the oven for 8–10 minutes, until the fish flakes easily.

Place the sliced cucumber, ginger and radish in a small bowl and sprinkle over the vinegar and sesame seeds. Set aside while the cod cooks.

Meanwhile, steam the vegetables for 1–2 minutes, until the spinach has wilted and the asparagus is tender.

Serve the cod on a bed of the steamed vegetables and top with the pickles.

White fish with tangy watercress sauce
Serves 2

2 cod, haddock or pollack
    fillets, approximately
    150 g (5 oz) each
2 tsp olive oil

For the sauce:
bunch of watercress
    (about 100 g/3½ oz)
handful of flat-leaf parsley
handful of basil leaves

1 tsp olive oil
large squeeze of lemon juice
1 tbsp water

SERVINGS		NUTRITIONAL INFO	
Protein	2½	Calories	184
Fat	½	Carbohydrate	1 g
Dairy	0	Protein	30 g
Fruit	0	Fibre	2 g
Vegetables	1	Salt	0.3 g

Make the sauce first. Strip off the watercress leaves, discarding the thickest parts of the stalks and any yellow leaves. Put the leaves in a large jug or liquidiser. Add the parsley and basil leaves, the olive oil and a squeeze of lemon juice. If using a hand blender, pulse the leaves together for a few seconds and then add a little water; if you are using a liquidiser, add some water at the start. Blend until the leaves are thoroughly chopped and there are no large pieces remaining, then pour into a small bowl.

To cook the fish: pat the fillets dry with kitchen paper. Using a non-stick frying pan, heat the olive oil over a medium to low heat. When the oil is hot, add the fish fillets, skin side down. Cook the fillets for 3–5 minutes, depending on how thick they are, then carefully turn over and cook for a little longer until done. The total cooking time should be 5–10 minutes, and the fish is ready when it flakes easily, revealing opaque flesh. Serve immediately, accompanied by some of the sauce (if you have made the sauce in a liquidiser, you may need to drain off some excess liquid first).

Tips:

▶ This dish can be made with any round white fish, and the sauce also goes well with oily fish such as salmon.

▶ On unrestricted days you could serve this with new potatoes.

Prawn and vegetable kebabs

Serves 1

150 g (5 oz) raw king
  prawns
7 cherry tomatoes
10 button mushrooms
½ courgette, sliced into rings
green salad leaves

SERVINGS		NUTRITIONAL INFO	
Protein	3	Calories	215
Fat	1	Carbohydrate	5 g
Dairy	0	Protein	31 g
Fruit	0	Fibre	3 g
Vegetables	3	Salt	0.8 g

For the marinade:
small handful of coriander
  leaves
½–1 green chilli (to taste),
  deseeded

2 tsp olive oil
2 tsp lemon or lime juice
black pepper

First make the marinade. Very finely chop the coriander leaves and the green chilli and transfer them to a bowl. Add the oil and lemon juice, and a good grinding of black pepper. Rinse the prawns, drain them well and add them to the marinade. Stir everything together, cover the bowl and put it to one side for 30 minutes. If using bamboo skewers, put them in to soak.

Thread the skewers, shaking excess marinade off the prawns as you lift them out of the bowl, and alternating them with the tomatoes, mushrooms and slices of courgette (discard what remains of the marinade). Preheat the grill to a very high heat, then lower it slightly and put the skewers under the heat – suspend them over a baking dish or roasting tin – for 5–6 minutes until they begin to brown and crisp nicely, turning them during this time. Serve the kebabs as soon as they are ready, with a green salad.

Black pepper salmon with olives and tomatoes
Serves 1

10 black olives, stoned and
    quartered
7 cherry tomatoes, halved
1 tsp olive oil
1 salmon fillet,
    skin removed, about
    120 g (4 oz)
black pepper
handful of basil leaves

SERVINGS		NUTRITIONAL INFO	
Protein	4	Calories	299
Fat	1½	Carbohydrate	6 g
Dairy	0	Protein	26 g
Fruit	0	Fibre	4 g
Vegetables	1	Salt	0.6 g

To serve:
small handful of rocket leaves
balsamic vinegar

Prepare the olives (if they have been in brine, rinse them well first) and put them in a bowl. Add the halved cherry tomatoes to the bowl as well, then add half a teaspoon of olive oil and stir them together.

Pat the salmon fillet dry with kitchen paper. Put the remaining oil on a plate and grind over lots of black pepper, then rub all sides of the salmon fillet in the oil-and-pepper mix.

Empty the olive-and-tomato mixture into a small non-stick pan over a low heat – they should just warm through rather than simmer or boil. Keep an eye on the pan to make sure the mixture isn't starting to burn, and take it off the heat if there is any sign that this might be happening; cover it to keep the mixture warm.

Preheat a ridged griddle pan or a small non-stick frying pan over a high heat. When the pan is really hot, put the salmon in the pan. Turn it over after 3 minutes and cook another side for a couple more minutes, then turn it again and repeat until cooked (the flesh should be completely opaque) and the edges are crisping up. Just before it is ready, add some torn basil leaves to the tomato and olives so that they wilt a little in the warmth of the pan.

Put the salmon fillet on a serving plate, and spoon the warm tomato, olive and basil mixture beside it. Accompany with a handful of rocket leaves drizzled with a little balsamic vinegar.

Fresh tuna steak with tomato salsa
Serves 1

1 tsp olive oil
1 fresh tuna steak, about
    150 g (5 oz)
black pepper

For the salsa:
1 medium tomato
3 spring onions, white only,
    finely chopped
1 tsp extra-virgin olive oil
squeeze of lemon juice
black pepper

small handful of basil leaves

To serve:
Salad leaves or a portion of
    steamed vegetables

SERVINGS		NUTRITIONAL INFO	
Protein	5	Calories	288
Fat	1	Carbohydrate	5 g
Dairy	0	Protein	37 g
Fruit	0	Fibre	3 g
Vegetables	1½	Salt	0.2 g

Make the salsa first. Cut the tomato into quarters, then finely chop the flesh into small cubes and put in a small bowl. Add the chopped spring onions to the chopped tomatoes, then the olive oil and lemon juice. Stir the salsa and add black pepper. Cover the bowl and set it to one side for 20 minutes. When ready to serve, tear the basil leaves and stir them into the salsa.

To cook the tuna, put the oil in a small non-stick frying pan over a high heat. Sprinkle both sides of the tuna steak very lightly with a little black pepper, then put in the pan when the oil is really hot and almost smoking. Cook it for no more than 2 minutes before turning it over and cooking the other side. How long this takes will depend on how thick the steak is; check by making a small cut in the middle of the steak with a sharp knife. Part the cut slightly and see how pink it is inside. Tuna is best eaten rare, like a beef steak, and should be slightly pink; cook it to taste but be careful not to overcook it or it will be tough and chewy. Put the tuna steak on a serving plate and spoon over the salsa. Accompany with a bowl of salad leaves or a portion of steamed vegetables.

Tips:

▶ As an alternative, use halibut of the same weight if you would rather not use tuna. Be careful to test that it is cooked and it may take a little more oil as well.

▶ Add some finely chopped red chilli and a little crushed garlic to the salsa for an extra kick.

Garlic prawns
Serves 1

1 tsp olive oil
1 garlic clove, crushed
180 g (6 oz) raw king
    prawns
juice of 1 lemon
½–1 tsp paprika (to taste)

SERVINGS		NUTRITIONAL INFO	
Protein	4	Calories	178
Fat	½	Carbohydrate	3 g
Dairy	0	Protein	32 g
Fruit	0	Fibre	1 g
Vegetables	1	Salt	0.8 g

To serve:
iceberg lettuce leaves

Put the oil in a non-stick frying pan over a very high heat. Add the garlic and cook very briefly, stirring it around so that it does not burn. Then immediately add the prawns and stir them in; cook them for a minute. Pour the lemon juice into the pan and add the paprika. Cook, stirring all the time, until the lemon juice has been taken up completely and the prawns are pink – this should take no longer than two minutes.

Serve immediately, spooning the prawns over iceberg lettuce leaves and wrapping them up as you eat.

Tips:

▶ This delicious Mediterranean dish can be adapted for unrestricted days. Add more lemon juice and cook it at a slightly lower temperature so that the prawns are cooked but there is still plenty of lemony, spicy sauce. Serve over rice instead of using the lettuce leaves.

▶ If you're using cooked prawns instead of raw ones, add the lemon juice and paprika immediately after putting the prawns in the pan.

Grilled plaice with a courgette nest

Serves 1

1 plaice fillet, about 180 g (6 oz)
drop of olive oil
1 tsp olive oil spread
1 small green courgette
1 tbsp low- or no-fat Greek
* yoghurt*
zest and juice of half a lemon
black pepper

SERVINGS		NUTRITIONAL INFO	
Protein	3	Calories	209
Fat	1	Carbohydrate	5 g
Dairy	½	Protein	30 g
Fruit	0	Fibre	1 g
Vegetables	2	Salt	0.6 g

Preheat the grill, and put a piece of foil large enough to hold the plaice fillet onto it. Lightly brush the oil onto the foil. Carefully lift the plaice onto the foil, skin side down, and dot it with the olive oil spread.

While the grill is heating, wipe the courgette and peel it into fine strips with a potato peeler, then set these to one side. Put the yoghurt into a small bowl and add some lemon zest and a very little of the juice. Stir the yoghurt and lemon together well. Put a pan of water on to boil.

While waiting for the pan to boil slide the plaice in the grill pan under the heat, but not too close (ideally, about 10 cm/4 in away) and cook the fish for about 5–6 minutes, until the flesh is opaque and the edges are beginning to crisp a little.

After the fish has been cooking for a couple of minutes, put the courgette ribbons into the boiling water and turn off the heat immediately. Leave them in the boiling water for no more than a minute, then drain them well. Add the courgette ribbons to the lemony yoghurt bowl, then quickly twist the ribbons into a nest with a fork, rather like spaghetti. Spoon the nest onto a serving plate and then add the cooked plaice, lifting it very carefully from the foil with a fish slice or similar flat utensil. Add a little black pepper and serve immediately.

Baked stuffed mackerel
Serves 2

*2 fresh mackerel, gutted
and heads removed,
about 200 g (7 oz) each
black pepper
several sprigs of thyme*

SERVINGS		NUTRITIONAL INFO	
Protein	7	Calories	270
Fat	0	Carbohydrate	1 g
Dairy	0	Protein	23 g
Fruit	0	Fibre	< 1 g
Vegetables	0	Salt	0.2 g

½ lemon, sliced
1 tbsp lemon juice

½ red onion, sliced
(for flavour only)

Preheat the oven to 200°C/400°F/Gas Mark 6. Tear off a large piece of foil and find an ovenproof dish big enough to hold the fish easily.

Place the fish in the middle of the sheet of foil. Season them, both inside and out, with lots of black pepper. Push the thyme into the cavities of the fish, then stuff them further with the slices of lemon and red onion. Bring the foil up around the two fish and add the lemon juice. Then fold the foil over the fish, make a parcel and seal it tightly.

Carefully lift the parcel into the ovenproof dish and put it in the hot oven. Bake the mackerel for 25 minutes then unwrap the parcel carefully, as steam will escape. Remove most of the stuffing, lift the fish onto plates and serve immediately. (If you like, you can quickly remove the skin from the fish and lift off the fillets first.) Serve with a green salad or steamed spinach.

Chicken and turkey

Roast chicken Provençal tray bake
Serves 1

1 chicken skinless breast,
weighing approximately
120 g (4 oz), chopped into
bite-sized pieces
¼ tsp olive oil
½ tsp balsamic vinegar

SERVINGS		NUTRITIONAL INFO	
Protein	4	Calories	197
Fat	0	Carbohydrate	8 g
Dairy	0	Protein	32 g
Fruit	0	Fibre	6 g
Vegetables	2½	Salt	0.4 g

2 garlic cloves, skins left on
   and crushed with the back
   of a knife
7 cherry tomatoes, sliced in
   half
1 leek, diced

1 tsp capers, drained
½ tsp dried oregano
half lemon
black pepper
40 g (1½ oz) watercress,
   tough stalks removed

Preheat the oven to 200°C/400°F/Gas Mark 6.

Put all of the ingredients (apart from the watercress) in an ovenproof dish and toss to combine all of the flavours. Season with black pepper and roast in the oven for 20 minutes, until the chicken pieces are cooked through and the ingredients are golden. Squeeze over the juice of the roasted lemon and serve immediately with the watercress.

Cream cheese, sundried tomato and chive-stuffed chicken with griddled fennel and courgette

Serves 1

1 tbsp low-fat cream cheese
1 small garlic clove, crushed
2 sundried tomatoes, finely
   chopped
1 tsp finely chopped chives
black pepper
1 skinless chicken breast,
   weighing 120 g (4 oz)
½ tsp olive oil
zest of half a lemon
half a courgette, sliced
   vertically into half slices

SERVINGS		NUTRITIONAL INFO	
Protein	4	Calories	253
Fat	0	Carbohydrate	5 g
Dairy	1	Protein	33 g
Fruit	0	Fibre	2 g
Vegetables	3	Salt	0.8 g

40 g (1½ oz) fennel, sliced
   into ½ cm (⅛ in) slices

Preheat the oven to 180°C/350°F/Gas Mark 4.

Mix the cream cheese, garlic, sundried tomatoes and chives together in a small bowl. Season with black pepper. Make a 5 cm (2 in) incision in the thickest part of the side of the chicken breast, about 2.5 cm (1 in) deep. Using a teaspoon, feed the stuffing into the chicken breast and seal the meat back together using a cocktail stick. Transfer to a small oven-proof dish and bake in the oven for 20–25 minutes, until the chicken is completely cooked through and the juices run clear when the meat is cut in the thickest part.

While the chicken is cooking, heat a griddle pan over a high heat. Mix together the olive oil and lemon zest and brush over the vegetable slices – season with black pepper.

Griddle the vegetable slices for 1–2 minutes each side, until nicely charred. Remove from the griddle and serve with the chicken breast.

Larb Gai – Thai chicken salad

Serves 1

1 small garlic clove, crushed
100 g (3½ oz) chicken or
*   turkey mince*
50 ml (1¾ fl oz) low-salt
*   chicken or vegetable stock*
squeeze of lime juice
4 spring onions, trimmed,
*   two sliced and two finely*
*   chopped*
1 red chilli, deseeded and
*   finely chopped (or to taste)*

SERVINGS		NUTRITIONAL INFO	
Protein	3½	Calories	143
Fat	0	Carbohydrate	5 g
Dairy	0	Protein	26 g
Fruit	0	Fibre	3 g
Vegetables	1½	Salt	0.4 g

sprig of mint
handful of coriander leaves

whole iceberg lettuce leaves,
about 80 g (2¾ oz), to serve

Mix the crushed garlic with the mince. Heat the stock in a small pan over a high heat until it is bubbling well. Then add the mince. Stir it in and continue stirring until the stock has evaporated and the mince has cooked; this should only take about 3–4 minutes (be careful not to overcook the mince, or it will be tough).

Once cooked, put the mince into a bowl, then add the lime juice, spring onions and chilli. Stir well. Strip the leaves from the mint stalk and chop the leaves with the coriander leaves. Add the chopped leaves to the bowl and stir through, then check for seasoning.

Serve immediately, on iceberg lettuce leaves.

Griddled turkey steaks with garlic spinach
Serves 1

1 turkey steak, about 120 g
   (4 oz) total weight
½ tsp Dijon mustard
½ lemon
½ tsp olive oil
black pepper

SERVINGS		NUTRITIONAL INFO	
Protein	4	Calories	211
Fat	0	Carbohydrate	5 g
Dairy	0	Protein	35 g
Fruit	0	Fibre	6 g
Vegetables	2½	Salt	t1.2 g

For the spinach:
200 g (7 oz) fresh baby
   spinach leaves
1 garlic clove, crushed
   nutmeg, to taste (optional)

Prepare the spinach first. Wash and remove any long stems, then chop it very roughly. Put it in a pan with the crushed garlic.

Before cooking the turkey steak, first press it down with your hands, flattening it out more. Then spread half the mustard over one side, smoothing it in with a knife or your fingers; turn it over and spread the rest of the mustard on the other side. Cut a couple of slices off the lemon, set aside and then juice the rest.

Preheat a ridged griddle pan or large non-stick frying pan. If using a griddle pan, brush the oil quickly over the surface of the ridges, and if using a frying pan, swirl the oil around to spread it out.

Just before cooking the turkey, put the pan of spinach over a medium heat, and add a little grated nutmeg to it.

Just as the oil starts to smoke in your frying pan or griddle, put on the turkey steak. Cook it on one side for about 3 minutes, then turn over and cook the other side for roughly the same time; sprinkle the lemon juice over the surface as you turn it. While you cook the steak, give the spinach a stir as well.

Check the turkey steak is cooked right through, then drain the spinach thoroughly, check it for seasoning and put it on a serving plate. Lift the steak onto the plate, season with black pepper, and put the lemon slices on the side for squeezing over the meat. Serve immediately.

Tandoori-style chicken with a shredded salad
Serves 1

1 large chicken breast,
skin removed
(about 150 g/5 oz)

2 tbsp natural yoghurt
½ tsp garam masala
½ tsp turmeric

½ tsp paprika

¼ tsp cayenne pepper

To serve:

80 g (2¾ oz) iceberg lettuce,
   finely shredded

2 spring onions, finely
   shredded into strips

2 cm (½ in) piece of
   cucumber, peeled, deseeded
   and finely shredded

SERVINGS		NUTRITIONAL INFO	
Protein	5	Calories	240
Fat	0	Carbohydrate	8 g
Dairy	1	Protein	39 g
Fruit	0	Fibre	2 g
Vegetables	0	Salt	0.5 g

lemon juice, to taste

Take the chicken and pierce it in several places with a sharp knife. Put the yoghurt in a glass or ceramic bowl and add the spices, stirring them well together.

Put the chicken in the bowl and smear the yoghurt mixture over it, massaging the mixture into the pierced holes. Cover the bowl with clingfilm and leave it in the refrigerator for 8–12 hours or overnight; if prepared to this stage in the morning, the chicken will be perfect to cook in the evening.

Preheat the oven to 200°C/400°F/Gas Mark 6. Shake any excess yoghurt marinade off the chicken and discard it. Then put the chicken in a deep baking dish (it should be deeper than the chicken breast). Cover the dish with foil, making sure it isn't touching the chicken and bake for 20 minutes. Remove the foil and cook for a further 15–20 minutes, turning the breast over during this time. Test to see if it is done (the juices should run clear when the chicken is pierced).

Mix together the finely shredded iceberg lettuce, fine shreds of spring onion and cucumber in a bowl and squeeze some lemon juice over them. Add a little pepper and toss the salad once more. Serve immediately with the hot chicken.

Tips:

▶ The chicken doesn't have to be baked – you can always grill it instead. Protect your grill pan or oven with foil and remember to turn the chicken over as it cooks. How long it takes will depend on your grill as individual types vary.

▶ Served cold, this chicken makes a good addition to a packed lunch; just allow it to cool and then refrigerate until needed.

Garlic and thyme chicken livers with mushrooms and broccoli in a cream cheese sauce
Serves 1

120 g (4 oz) chicken livers
1 tbsp low-fat cream cheese
2 tbsp hot chicken stock
¼ tsp olive oil
2 spears tenderstem or
* purple-sprouting*
* broccoli, cut into*
* 2 cm (½ in) slices*
1 clove garlic, crushed
1 tsp thyme leaves, chopped

7 small chestnut mushrooms,
* sliced*
black pepper

SERVINGS		NUTRITIONAL INFO	
Protein	4	Calories	203
Fat	0	Carbohydrate	5 g
Dairy	1	Protein	31 g
Fruit	0	Fibre	4 g
Vegetables	1½	Salt	0.6 g

Begin by picking over the chicken livers, slicing off any bits of fat and sinew. Pat dry.

Mix the cream cheese with the chicken stock and set aside. Heat the oil in a frying pan over a medium heat. When the oil is hot, add the livers and the broccoli and fry for 2 minutes, until the livers have browned on all sides. Add the garlic, thyme and mushrooms and continue to fry for a further 2 minutes, until everything is nicely golden. Turn the heat down to low and pour in the cream cheese and stock mixture. Allow to bubble for 30 seconds before removing from the heat. Serve seasoned with lots of black pepper.

Chicken escalope with paprika and herbs
Serves 1

1 chicken breast, skin
    removed, about 150 g
    (5 oz)
1 tsp paprika
1 tsp dried mixed herbs
½ tsp olive oil

SERVINGS		NUTRITIONAL INFO	
Protein	5	Calories	199
Fat	0	Carbohydrate	3 g
Dairy	0	Protein	35 g
Fruit	0	Fibre	2 g
Vegetables	2	Salt	0.4 g

To serve:
bowlful of green salad, about
    60 g (2 oz)
handful of rocket leaves,
    about 20 g (2/3 oz)

6 radishes, trimmed and
    halved
2 lemon slices
black pepper

Tear off a large piece of greaseproof paper and fold it in half, then open it up. Remove any excess fat from the chicken and put it on one half of the paper; fold the other half on top of the chicken breast. Take a rolling pin or similar heavy item and whack the chicken breast, flattening it until it is no thicker than 1 cm (¼ in). Put the paprika and herbs on a plate and mix them together thoroughly.

Heat the oil in a small non-stick frying pan over a medium heat. When it is hot, take the chicken breast and dip one side into the spice and herb mix, then flip it over and do the other side. Put the chicken escalope into the frying pan and cook it for 3–4 minutes – the oil will spit, so you may want to use a splatter guard. Turn the escalope over and cook the other side for a further 3 minutes – hold it flat with a fish slice for the last minute or so.

While the chicken is cooking, put the salad together. Squeeze one of the lemon slices over the leaves and radishes, and mix everything together well. Check the chicken is done – the juices will run clear when it is – and lift it out of the pan. Blot it briefly on kitchen paper and put it on a warmed serving plate. Squeeze the other slice of lemon over it, grind a little black pepper on top and serve immediately with the salad on the side.

Tip:

▶ You could also use a turkey escalope in this dish and substitute other spices – try a Cajun spice mix, for example. Don't use too much, though, as it can burn easily and taste bitter.

Chicken or turkey stir-fry with mange tout and green beans
Serves 1

*1 small chicken breast, about
    100 g (3½ oz), skin
    removed, or turkey breast
    of the same weight
juice of half a lemon
1 tsp light soy sauce
25 g (¾ oz) mange tout,
    trimmed*

SERVINGS		NUTRITIONAL INFO	
Protein	3½	Calories	235
Fat	1	Carbohydrate	8 g
Dairy	0	Protein	30 g
Fruit	0	Fibre	6 g
Vegetables	2½	Salt	0.8 g

*50 g (1¾ oz) thin French
  beans, trimmed*
2 spears sprouting broccoli
*4 spring onions, sliced
  diagonally*
1 garlic clove, finely chopped

*2 cm (½ in) square piece of
  fresh ginger root, finely
  chopped*
*1 small red chilli, deseeded
  and finely chopped
  (optional)*
2 tsp rapeseed oil

Cut the chicken or turkey breast into strips, no wider than 1 cm (¼ in) and 6 cm (2⅓ in) in length. Put these in a bowl and add a teaspoon of the lemon juice and the soy sauce. Stir to coat, then cover the bowl with clingfilm and put it in the refrigerator for 30 minutes.

Prepare all the vegetables: chop the mange tout and beans into strips the same length as the chicken or turkey pieces; break up the spears of sprouting broccoli and cut off any woody stems; slice the spring onions diagonally and include some of the green part.

Use a non-stick wok or large non-stick frying pan. Put it on a high heat, add the oil and take the chicken or turkey strips out of the refrigerator. Using a slotted spoon, remove the meat from the marinade and put it into the wok – it should spit if the oil is hot enough, so be careful. Cook for about 3–4 minutes, stirring well until it begins to colour, and then remove the meat from the wok and set aside. Add the chopped vegetables, spring onions, garlic, ginger and chilli and cook them quickly until crisp but tender; stir them around or they will stick to the pan and burn. Return the meat and any juices to the wok, add the rest of the lemon juice and allow the chicken to heat up thoroughly, which will take another minute or two. Serve immediately.

Tangy chicken drumsticks with crudités and a harissa dip
Serves 1

*2 chicken drumsticks, skin
  removed, about 120 g
  (4 oz) each*

For the marinade:
2 spring onions, finely chopped
3 tbsp Worcester sauce
splash Tabasco sauce
black pepper
½ tsp cinnamon
½ tsp ground allspice
¼ tsp ground cumin
3 tsp cider vinegar

SERVINGS		NUTRITIONAL INFO	
Protein	5	Calories	282
Fat	0	Carbohydrate	12 g
Dairy	½	Protein	45 g
Fruit	0	Fibre	3 g
Vegetables	2½	Salt	1 g

For the crudités and dip:
3 celery sticks
3 spring onions
5 cm (2 in) piece of cucumber
2 tbsp low-fat Greek yoghurt
½ –1 tsp harissa (to taste)

Carefully remove the skin from the drumsticks. Mix all the marinade ingredients together in a small ceramic or glass dish just large enough to hold the two drumsticks. Put the drumsticks in and turn them in the marinade, then spoon some of the marinade over them. Cover with clingfilm and refrigerate for at least 6 hours, but for no longer than 12 hours.

Preheat the oven to 190°C/375°F/Gas Mark 5. Lift the chicken out of the marinade, then sieve the remainder of the marinade into a small baking dish (discard the spring onion left in the sieve). Add a tablespoon of water and the chicken drumsticks. Turn them over and over in the marinade and then put the baking dish in the oven. Cook for 35–40 minutes or until the drumsticks are done, which will depend on their size. Turn them over twice during this time.

Prepare the crudités and dip just before the drumsticks are ready. Trim the celery, removing the strings with a knife, and the spring onions. Peel the cucumber, cut it in half, remove the seeds and then slice it into strips. Spoon the yoghurt into a small bowl and gradually add the harissa, tasting it as you go along to make sure that you get the dip just as hot as you want it. Serve with the crudités as soon as the drumsticks are ready.

Tips:

▶ Instead of using individual spices in the marinade, you could use a teaspoon of jerk seasoning; it will taste different, but be equally good. If the brand you choose has a high proportion of chilli in it – they vary – don't use the Tabasco.

▶ The drumsticks can also be served cold.

Not-quite-coronation chicken
Serves 1

½ tsp garam masala

¼ tsp turmeric

2 tbsp low- or no-fat Greek yoghurt

1 tbsp low-fat mayonnaise

dash of Worcester sauce, to taste black pepper

150 g (5 oz) cooked chicken breast, skin and any excess fat removed

1 celery stick, trimmed

2 spring onions, trimmed

handful of lettuce leaves, about 60 g (2 oz)

handful of flaked almonds, about 10 g (⅓ oz)

SERVINGS		NUTRITIONAL INFO	
Protein	5	Calories	430
Fat	2	Carbohydrate	12 g
Dairy	½	Protein	56 g
Fruit	0	Fibre	3 g
Vegetables	½	Salt	1.3 g

Put a non-stick frying pan on a medium heat. When it is hot, spoon in the garam masala and turmeric and stir them around until they begin to smell toasted. As soon as they reach that stage, take the pan off the heat and tip the spices into a bowl.

Add the yoghurt and the mayonnaise to the bowl, and a small dash of Worcester sauce. Stir them together, then taste, and add more Worcester sauce if needed. Grind in some black pepper. Chop the chicken breast into chunks about 1.5 cm (½ in) square, and add these to the bowl. Stir everything together, cover the bowl with clingfilm and refrigerate for at least an hour, preferably two.

Pull the strings from the celery stick and chop it into small pieces, then chop one spring onion into diagonal slices and the other into finer pieces. Take the chicken out of the refrigerator, add the chopped celery and spring onion, and stir everything together. Put the salad leaves on a serving plate and spoon the chicken salad on top; scatter over the almonds and serve immediately.

Griddled chicken with Asian slaw and a quick sambal

Serves 1

Juice and zest of 1 lime
½ tsp dark soy sauce
1 skinless chicken breast,
*   weighing 120 g (4 oz)*
1½ tbsp shredded white cabbage
40 g (1½ oz) cos lettuce
*   leaves, roughly torn*
3 baby sweetcorn, sliced in
*   half vertically*

SERVINGS		NUTRITIONAL INFO	
Protein	4	Calories	170
Fat	0	Carbohydrate	6 g
Dairy	0	Protein	30 g
Fruit	0	Fibre	3 g
Vegetables	1½	Salt	0.7 g

1 tbsp coriander, chopped
1 cm (¼ in) piece of ginger,
    finely grated

For the sambal:
1 red chilli, finely chopped
½ garlic clove, crushed
squeeze of lime juice

Drizzle half the lime juice, zest and the soy sauce over the chicken and set aside in the fridge for a minimum of 1 hour, up to overnight.

Heat a griddle pan over a medium heat. When smoking hot, add the chicken breast and griddle for 4 minutes on each side. Check that the chicken is cooked by inserting a skewer into the thickest part of the meat – if the juices run clear, set the chicken breast aside. Griddle for a further 2–3 minutes, if necessary.

Meanwhile, toss the cabbage, lettuce, sweetcorn and coriander in the ginger and remaining lime juice and zest and set aside.

To make the sambal, mince the ingredients in a pestle and mortar until they form a thick, homogenous paste.

Serve the chicken with the slaw and the sambal. The chicken can be served hot or cold.

Meat dishes

Grilled lamb, aubergine and sundried tomato stack
Serves 1

1 tsp tomato purée
1 garlic clove, crushed
¼ tsp olive oil
¼ tsp fennel seeds, crushed
    with a pestle and mortar

SERVINGS		NUTRITIONAL INFO	
Protein	4	Calories	280
Fat	0	Carbohydrate	6 g
Dairy	0	Protein	27 g
Fruit	0	Fibre	5 g
Vegetables	1½	Salt	0.5 g

120 g (4 oz) lamb loin,
sliced into 1 cm (¼ in)
slices
⅓ medium aubergine,
sliced into 1 cm (¼ in)
slices

2 sundried tomatoes,
chopped
small handful of basil leaves
½ tsp balsamic vinegar
black pepper

Mix together the tomato purée, garlic and olive oil and fennel seeds and brush over the lamb and aubergine. Preheat a griddle pan over a high heat and when smoking hot, griddle the lamb and aubergine slices for 1 minute each side. Remove from the pan and layer the slices up on a plate, sprinkling with the sundried tomato and basil. Finish by drizzling over the balsamic vinegar and seasoning with black pepper.

Harissa-roasted pork fillet with pumpkin and tomatoes

Serves 1

½ tsp caraway seeds
¼ tsp coriander seeds
½ tsp paprika
1 red chilli
1 garlic clove
¼ tsp olive oil
120 g (4 oz) pork fillet, sinew
and fatty bits sliced off
80 g (2¾ oz) pumpkin,
chopped into 1 cm
(¼ in) dice

1 medium tomato, sliced into
quarters
1 tsp lemon juice
1 tbsp coriander, chopped

SERVINGS		NUTRITIONAL INFO	
Protein	4	Calories	175
Fat	0	Carbohydrate	5 g
Dairy	0	Protein	31 g
Fruit	0	Fibre	6 g
Vegetables	2	Salt	0.2 g

Toast the caraway seeds, coriander seeds and paprika in a small frying pan for 1 minute, until fragrant.

To make the harissa, mince the chilli, garlic, toasted spices and olive oil in a pestle and mortar until they make a paste. Rub the harissa over the pork fillet until completely covered. Set aside in the fridge for a minimum of 2 hours, up to overnight.

Preheat the oven to 190°C/375°F/Gas Mark 5.

Transfer the pork fillet to an ovenproof dish, add the pumpkin and tomatoes to the dish and toss together so that everything is coated in a little harissa.

Roast in the oven for 15–20 minutes, until the juices of the fillet run clear when pierced with a skewer. Drizzle over the lemon juice, sprinkle over the coriander and serve immediately.

Lamb chops and 'little dishes'
Serves 1

2 small lamb chops or cutlets
(about 120 g/4 oz)
1 tsp olive oil
¼ tsp paprika
pinch of turmeric
pinch of cayenne
handful of mint leaves,
*   finely chopped*
2 sprigs of rosemary

SERVINGS		NUTRITIONAL INFO	
Protein	4	Calories	383
Fat	1½	Carbohydrate	7 g
Dairy	0	Protein	38 g
Fruit	0	Fibre	3 g
Vegetables	3	Salt	0.6 g

For the 'little dishes':
5 cm (2 in) piece of
*   cucumber, peeled and*
*   finely sliced*

6 large green olives
handful of salad leaves,
*   about 60 g (2 oz)*

7 cherry tomatoes, sliced
1 tsp olive oil
squeeze of lemon juice

1 tsp balsamic vinegar
½ red chilli (optional), finely
sliced

You will need a ceramic or glass ovenproof dish. Pat the chops dry and remove any excess fat; if you are using cutlets, strip the fat from the bone.

Put the olive oil in the bottom of the ovenproof dish and add the paprika, turmeric and cayenne, along with the chopped mint leaves and the whole rosemary sprigs. Mix everything together and then add the chops. Move them about to coat them in the oil and spice mix, then turn the chops over so that the other side is coated with the mixture as well. Cover the dish with clingfilm and leave it in the refrigerator for an hour.

Near the end of that time, preheat the oven to 200°C/ 400°F/Gas Mark 6 and start to prepare the 'little dishes'. Peel the cucumber, slice it very thinly, then set aside.

Take the clingfilm off the ovenproof dish and put it in the oven. Cook the lamb for approximately 6 minutes, and then turn the chops over and cook for another 6 minutes, or until the lamb is done to your liking (exactly how long will depend on the thickness of the meat and personal taste).

While the lamb is cooking, finish the accompaniments. Put the olives in a little dish – rinse them first if they have been in brine. Put the salad leaves in a bowl. Scatter the sliced cherry tomatoes over the salad leaves. Dress the salad by drizzling over the olive oil, toss, then add a squeeze of lemon juice. Rinse the cucumber slices and put these in another small dish, add the balsamic vinegar and stir. Very finely slice some red chilli and scatter over the cucumber slices.

As soon as the meat is ready, lift it out of the ovenproof dish on to a serving plate. Serve, surrounded by the 'little dishes'.

Tip

▶ If you're not fond of lamb, substitute chicken breast, but note
that it will take much longer to cook so adjust the timings
accordingly. It could also be grilled rather than roasted, as
could the lamb chops.

Vegetarian mains

Quick cauliflower and okra curry with a yoghurt and mint raita
Serves 1

½ tsp olive oil

2 spring onions, sliced

1 garlic clove, crushed

2 cm (½ in) piece of ginger,
    finely grated

½ tsp ground cumin seeds

½ tsp ground coriander seeds

¼ tsp garam masala

¼ tsp hot chilli powder

¼ tsp black mustard seeds
    (optional)

4 cauliflower florets
    (40 g/1½ oz)

½ tin chopped tomatoes

8 small okra

1 tbsp chopped coriander

For the raita:

3 tbsp fat-free natural
    yoghurt

2½ cm (1 in) piece of
    cucumber, coarsely grated

1 tsp finely chopped mint

SERVINGS		NUTRITIONAL INFO	
Protein	0	Calories	106
Fat	0	Carbohydrate	13 g
Dairy	1	Protein	7 g
Fruit	0	Fibre	7 g
Vegetables	2½	Salt	0.2 g

Heat the oil in a small medium frying pan over a medium heat.
When the oil is hot, add the spring onions and fry gently for

2–3 minutes, until softened and golden. Add the garlic, ginger, spices and cauliflower and fry for a further 1 or 2 minutes, until fragrant and the cauliflower is golden. Add the tomatoes and simmer for 3–4 minutes, until the sauce has thickened and reduced slightly. Add the okra and cook for a further 2 minutes, until slightly softened.

Meanwhile, mix together the yoghurt, cucumber and mint to make the raita. Serve the curry sprinkled with the coriander and the raita on the side.

Ginger, soy and chilli tofu skewers with Chinese leaf and mange tout salad
Serves 1

125 g (4⅓ oz) (half a pack)
  firm tofu
2 tsp low-salt soy sauce
¼ tsp sesame oil
¼ tsp crushed chilli flakes
2 cm (½ in) piece of root
  ginger, finely grated

SERVINGS		NUTRITIONAL INFO	
Protein	2½	Calories	151
Fat	0	Carbohydrate	8 g
Dairy	0	Protein	15 g
Fruit	0	Fibre	4 g
Vegetables	2	Salt	1.8 g

For the salad:
⅕ of a head of Chinese leaves,
  finely sliced
80 g (2¾ oz) mange tout,
  sliced in half lengthways

½ red chilli, finely chopped
juice of half a lime
½ lemongrass stalk, woody
  outer layers removed and
  finely sliced

For the skewers, slice the tofu into long strips, approximately 10 cm (4 in) long and 2.5 cm (1 in) wide and thread onto wooden skewers. Transfer the skewers into a baking tray, mix together the soy sauce, sesame oil, chilli flakes and ginger and pour over the skewers. Set aside to marinate for up to an hour, turning the skewers over occasionally to marinate evenly.

Meanwhile, mix together the chilli, lime juice and lemongrass for the dressing.

Preheat the grill to high and grill the skewers for 1–2 minutes each side, until browned.

Toss the salad in the dressing and serve with the skewers and any juices left in the grill pan.

Italian bean stew
Serves 2

1 x 227 g (7½ oz) tin
    whole or chopped plum
    tomatoes
1 tsp olive oil
1 leek, trimmed
    and chopped
1 celery stick, chopped
2 garlic cloves, chopped
1 tsp dried mixed herbs,
    Italian if available
160 g (5½ oz) curly kale
    or Savoy cabbage leaves,
    finely chopped

120 g (4 oz) frozen soya
    beans
black pepper

SERVINGS		NUTRITIONAL INFO	
Protein	1	Calories	172
Fat	0	Carbohydrate	11 g
Dairy	0	Protein	14 g
Fruit	0	Fibre	9 g
Vegetables	2½	Salt	0.2 g

Drain the tin of tomatoes over a bowl and set aside the juice. Put a pan over a medium heat and add the oil. Once hot, add the leek and celery and cook them gently, stirring, until they start to soften; don't let them burn. Add the garlic, stir it in and cook for a further minute. Then add the tomatoes, breaking them up as you stir them in, and a sprinkling of the mixed herbs.

Cook very gently for a further 8–10 minutes, stirring regularly, until everything is really tender. Keep an eye on the pan, and if it looks as though the mixture is sticking to the bottom, lower the temperature and add a splash of water.

Now add the chopped kale or cabbage and the juice from the tomatoes, and simmer for 15 minutes or so until the kale is thoroughly cooked; again, if it looks as though the liquid may be evaporating too quickly, add a little more water. Finally, add the frozen soya beans and cook the stew for 7–8 minutes, or until the beans are soft but not mushy; adjust the heat if necessary so that you end up with a stew and not a soup (see the tip below). Check the seasoning, add a little black pepper, and serve immediately.

Tip:

▶ This recipe also makes a great thick and chunky soup – just rinse out the tomato tin with water and add that water to the pan to increase the amount of liquid.

▶ Stew or soup, this dish freezes beautifully, and a little grated cheese (such as Edam) is delicious on top.

Mint, feta and soya bean salad
Serves 1

*60 g (2 oz) frozen soya beans
or fresh edamame
1 tsp olive oil
½ tsp balsamic vinegar*

*¼ tsp Dijon or wholegrain
mustard
2 celery sticks, strings removed
and finely chopped*

6 spring onions,
  chopped
2 cm (½ in) piece
  of cucumber
2 sprigs of fresh mint,
  leaves removed
30 g (1 oz) feta cheese

SERVINGS		NUTRITIONAL INFO	
Protein	1	Calories	220
Fat	½	Carbohydrate	8 g
Dairy	1	Protein	16 g
Fruit	0	Fibre	7 g
Vegetables	2½	Salt	1.4 g

To serve:
handful of lettuce leaves,   *black pepper*
  about 60 g (2 oz)

Bring a pan of water to the boil and add the frozen soya beans. Return to the boil, then lower the heat and simmer until tender, about 7–8 minutes. Test the beans as they cook and be careful not to overdo them – not only do they go mushy, they also lose their attractive bright-green colour. Cook fresh edamame for a shorter time, until warm and tender. Once cooked, drain and set aside.

Put the oil, vinegar and mustard in a large bowl, beat them together until the mustard is dissolved, and add the warm beans. Stir them well and set the bowl to one side.

Prepare the rest of the ingredients: chop the celery and spring onions; partly peel the cucumber along its length, making stripes, then cut in half, remove the seeds and cut the halves across into semi-circles. Take the mint leaves, roll them up and chop them into fine strips. Put all the chopped vegetables and the mint into the bowl with the soya beans, and stir everything together well.

Rinse the feta under running water to get rid of any excess brine.

Put the lettuce leaves on a serving plate, and spoon over the fresh bean salad. Then crumble the feta over the top and add a generous amount of black pepper. Serve immediately.

Baked eggs, Tunisian style
Serves 1

1 tsp olive oil
½ green pepper, deseeded and chopped
½ leek, sliced into rings (about 80 g/2¾ oz)
1 garlic clove, finely chopped
½ yellow courgette (green if unavailable), sliced into rings
1 medium tomato, deseeded and chopped
½ tsp paprika

¼–½ tsp cayenne pepper, to taste
dash of wine vinegar
black pepper
2 eggs

SERVINGS		NUTRITIONAL INFO	
Protein	2	Calories	265
Fat	½	Carbohydrate	9 g
Dairy	0	Protein	19 g
Fruit	0	Fibre	6 g
Vegetables	3½	Salt	0.5 g

Preheat the oven to 200°C/400°F/Gas Mark 6.

Heat the oil in a pan over a medium heat, then add the pepper and cook gently for a couple of minutes. Then add the leek and garlic and cook the mixture gently for another 5–10 minutes, stirring so that it doesn't burn (cover the pan if you wish, but don't forget to check it). Then add the courgette, tomato, paprika and cayenne pepper. Add a dash of vinegar and plenty of black pepper, and cook the mixture for another 5 minutes. Meanwhile find a small ovenproof dish that can also be taken to the table and warm it in the oven.

Spoon the vegetable mixture into the warmed ovenproof dish and make two depressions in the surface of the mixture with the back of a ladle or a wooden spoon; don't press right through to the surface of the dish. (If there isn't room for two separate depressions, make a single larger one in the middle.) Break the eggs, one by one, into a cup and slide them into these dips. Put the dish into the oven and bake until the eggs are just set – the yolks should be runny and the whites set – which will take about 8 minutes. Serve immediately, straight from the dish.

Stuffed Portobello mushrooms
Serves 1

2 large Portobello mushrooms, about 150 g (5 oz) in total, wiped
100 g (3½ oz) fresh spinach leaves, washed, stringy stalks removed, and chopped
4 walnut halves (optional), roughly chopped
black pepper
30 g (1 oz) low-fat mozzarella

1 tsp good-quality pesto
scant tsp balsamic vinegar

To serve:
handful of salad leaves, about 60 g (2 oz)

SERVINGS		NUTRITIONAL INFO	
Protein	0	Calories	234
Fat	2	Carbohydrate	3 g
Dairy	1	Protein	15 g
Fruit	0	Fibre	5 g
Vegetables	4	Salt	0.6 g

Preheat the oven to 200°C/400°F/Gas Mark 6. Use a small ovenproof dish just big enough to hold the mushrooms without them tipping over, and line it with foil. Wipe the mushrooms (only peel them if necessary). Trim the stalks so that the interior is flattish and put them in the dish, stalk side uppermost. Put the dish in the oven and bake the mushrooms for 15 minutes.

Towards the end of this time, put the washed and prepared spinach in a pan over a medium heat; there's no need to add any extra water. Wilt it down until it is hugely reduced in volume, stirring regularly to make sure it doesn't stick – this will only take about 2–3 minutes.

Drain the spinach well, pressing it down in the sieve to get as much liquid out as possible. Empty it out onto a chopping board and chop it again, even more finely. Add the roughly chopped walnuts to the spinach, along with plenty of black pepper and mix them in. Cut the mozzarella into small pieces and set it aside.

Take the mushrooms out of the oven. Carefully spread a teaspoon of pesto over each one, then divide the spinach and walnut mixture between them. Scatter the pieces of mozzarella on top and return the dish to the oven for 5–6 minutes, until the mozzarella is beginning to spread and colour up.

Put the stuffed mushrooms on a plate and drizzle a little balsamic vinegar across the surface. Serve immediately, accompanied by a side dish of salad leaves

Tip:

▶ Buy a good quality pesto; it's worth it. Less expensive varieties often contain cheaper oils than pure olive oil, and cashews rather than pine nuts. Some are even padded out with potato flakes and sugar, so check the ingredients list carefully.

Roasted vegetables with grilled halloumi
Serves 1

1 slice from a small
   pumpkin, about 80 g
   (2¾ oz)
½ small aubergine, about
   80 g (2¾ oz) in weight
½ green pepper
1 tsp olive oil
½ large courgette, chopped

SERVINGS		NUTRITIONAL INFO	
Protein	0	Calories	233
Fat	0	Carbohydrate	6 g
Dairy	1½	Protein	15 g
Fruit	0	Fibre	4 g
Vegetables	4	Salt	0.8 g

For the halloumi:
50 g (1¾ oz) low-fat or light
   halloumi, sliced
pinch or two of dried thyme
   or oregano

½ tsp olive oil
handful of fresh oregano
   (optional)

Preheat the oven to 200°C/400°F/Gas Mark 6. Peel the piece of pumpkin and discard any seeds and stringy bits. Cut the firm flesh into chunks of about 1.5 cm (½ in) (you should have about 3 heaped tablespoons). Chop the aubergine and pepper into pieces about the same size. Put the teaspoon of olive oil into a small roasting tin or ovenproof dish and pop it in the oven to warm through. When it is warm, tip the dish so that the oil runs across it, then add the pumpkin, aubergine and pepper. Spread them out, turning each piece in the oil, and put the dish back in the oven for 15 minutes. Then stir the vegetables again and add the chopped courgette. Return the dish to the oven for a further 10 minutes, and check the vegetables for softness – they may take a further 5 minutes or so, depending on the variety of pumpkin used.

When the vegetables are nearly ready, prepare the halloumi. If you have a separate grill and oven, preheat the grill, brush the slices with the oil and rub the herbs into them. Pop the slices on foil and grill both sides.

If your oven and grill are combined, preheat a small non-stick frying pan. Sprinkle both sides of the halloumi slices with a little dried thyme or oregano and add the half-teaspoon of olive oil to the pan. When the pan is hot, fry the halloumi quickly for about a minute on each side.

Put the vegetables on a serving plate, and carefully lift the halloumi beside them. Scatter the fresh oregano over everything, if using, and serve immediately.

Tip:

▶ If you can't find low-fat halloumi you can use low-fat mozzarella instead, but treat it a little differently. Once the roasted vegetables are tender, scatter 50 g (1¾ oz) chopped mozzarella on top; pop the dish under a hot grill until the mozzarella has melted and serve immediately.

Fluffy omelette with spring onions
Serves 1

2 eggs
black pepper
a little sunflower spread
3 large spring onions,
    trimmed and finely
    chopped
10 g (⅓ oz) low-fat
    Cheddar cheese, grated

SERVINGS		NUTRITIONAL INFO	
Protein	2	Calories	258
Fat	0	Carbohydrate	1 g
Dairy	½	Protein	21 g
Fruit	0	Fibre	1 g
Vegetables	1½	Salt	0.7 g

To garnish:
handful of watercress, about 80 g (2¾ oz)

Carefully separate the eggs into yolks and whites and put them in two separate bowls. Beat the yolks, adding a little black pepper to them. Whisk the whites – an electric whisk makes this easier – until they stand in soft peaks. Then carefully fold them into the beaten yolks, bit by bit.

Melt the sunflower spread in a small non-stick frying pan over a low to medium heat. Pour in the egg mixture and level the surface off with a palette knife, fish slice or similar flat utensil. Then scatter the spring onions over it, and finally add the grated cheese. Cook the omelette for 4–5 minutes, by which time the top should be fluffy and warm and the underside (when you lift it up slightly with your knife or fish slice) golden brown. Slide it onto a serving plate, allowing it to fold over slightly as you do so, and garnish with the watercress. Serve immediately.

'Almost a celeri remoulade'
Serves 1

150 g (5 oz) untrimmed
  celeriac
3 celery sticks

For the dressing:
½ tsp Dijon mustard
1 tbsp low-fat mayonnaise
1 tsp capers
black pepper

SERVINGS		NUTRITIONAL INFO	
Protein	0	Calories	148
Fat	1	Carbohydrate	9 g
Dairy	0	Protein	4 g
Fruit	0	Fibre	5 g
Vegetables	4	Salt	1.6 g

To serve:
handful of iceberg lettuce leaves, about 80 g (2¾ oz)

Make the dressing first. Put the mustard and the mayonnaise in a large bowl. Rinse the capers (they are generally sold in brine), chop them roughly, then add them to the bowl as well. Stir everything together, adding black pepper to taste.

Put a pan of water on to boil. Trim the celeriac and cut into thin pieces about 3 cm (1 in) long wherever possible, and then cut these pieces into fine matchsticks.

Once all the celeriac is ready, carefully slide the strips into the pan of rapidly boiling water. Return the pan to the boil and cook the celeriac for just one minute, then drain the celeriac in a sieve. Rinse it immediately under a cold tap and shake it well to dry it thoroughly (if necessary, pat dry in a clean tea towel or with kitchen paper).

While it is drying off, prepare the celery sticks. Pull off any strings, then slice them in two down the length of the sticks and then very finely slice across. Put these into the bowl with the dressing, and then add the cool celeriac. Mix everything carefully, ensuring all the celeriac and celery is coated with the dressing, then cover the bowl with clingfilm and refrigerate for an hour.

Serve with scoops made from iceberg lettuce leaves.

Tip:

▶ This is also good served with a chicken breast or a salmon fillet (see page 276, 'Baked chicken with rosemary', or page 200, 'Salmon parcels with aromatic salad' for ideas).

Oriental vegetable stir-fry with marinated tofu and cashews

Serves 1

150 g (5 oz) firm tofu
juice of 1 lemon
1 tsp light soy sauce
1 small pak choi
*   or half a large*
*   one, trimmed (about*
*   60 g/2 oz)*
6 spring onions
1 large garlic clove, finely
*   chopped*
1–2 cm (¼–½ in) piece of
*   fresh ginger root, finely*
*   chopped*

2 tsp rapeseed or other
*   neutral-tasting vegetable*
*   oil*
2 handfuls of beansprouts –
*   about 4 tbsp*
1 tbsp cashew nuts

SERVINGS		NUTRITIONAL INFO	
Protein	2½	Calories	286
Fat	1½	Carbohydrate	12 g
Dairy	0	Protein	19 g
Fruit	0	Fibre	6 g
Vegetables	2½	Salt	0.6 g

Carefully cut the block of tofu into slices about 1 cm (¼ in) thick. Put the lemon juice and soy sauce in a dish and blend them together. Spread out a double thickness of kitchen paper, then gently lift the first slice of tofu onto the kitchen paper, fold the paper over and lightly press down on the tofu to blot it. Peel the paper back and then carefully lift the tofu slice into the dish with the marinade. Repeat with the other slices, and then spoon a little of the marinade over the tofu pieces. Cover and leave for 10 minutes, then very carefully turn the slices over. Leave for a further 10 minutes.

Take the pak choi and slice the leaf part into very fine strips then push to one side while you cut the stems into broader pieces. Chop the spring onions diagonally across, including some of the green part. Set these aside with the chopped garlic and ginger.

Heat the oil in a non-stick wok or large non-stick frying pan until it is hot. Get some more kitchen paper, lift the tofu out of the marinade and blot it as before. Cut each slice in half, making rough squares, and gently lower them into the pan. Cook for 3 minutes, and then turn them over carefully. Take the wok off the heat while doing this so the remaining ones don't overcook, then return the wok to the heat and cook the other sides. Have a plate ready, and lift the pieces of tofu onto the plate with a spatula, again doing so with the wok off the heat.

Return the wok to the heat – enough oil should have remained in it – and add the spring onions, the pak choi stems, garlic and ginger. Cook and stir these for 3 minutes, then add the beansprouts and the pak choi leaf strips. Stir briefly, then add a tablespoon of the marinade and cook it off, stirring. Add the cashew nuts and stir the vegetables around, then carefully replace the tofu. Cook without stirring for a few more seconds, and then transfer the stir-fry to a warm plate. Serve immediately.

Tip:

▶ Tofu can be difficult to handle, but it is worth it; not only is it highly nutritious, tofu also takes up flavours beautifully.

Cauliflower and mushroom curry with yoghurt
Serves 2

1 small cauliflower (about 200 g/7 oz)
250 g (8⅔ oz) mushrooms
½ tsp cayenne pepper

½ tsp ground coriander
½ tsp ground cumin
½ tsp turmeric
½ tsp ground black pepper

2 tsp rapeseed or other
neutral-tasting
vegetable oil
250 ml (8½ fl oz) boiling
water
2 heaped tbsp natural yoghurt
handful of flaked almonds,
or a handful of coriander
leaves, chopped

SERVINGS		NUTRITIONAL INFO	
Protein	0	Calories	153
Fat	1	Carbohydrate	8 g
Dairy	1	Protein	10 g
Fruit	0	Fibre	5 g
Vegetables	3	Salt	0.1 g

Trim the cauliflower and break the florets into pieces no larger than 2 cm (½ in); clean and slice the mushrooms. Set the vegetables aside. Put all the spices and the black pepper in a small bowl and mix them together.

Put the oil in a large pan and warm it up over a medium heat. Once it is hot, add the spices and stir, frying them off for 1 minute. Add the mushrooms and the cauliflower florets and stir for another minute – don't stop stirring or they could stick to the pan.

Add the boiling water to the vegetables and bring the pan to a simmer. Cover and cook for 10 minutes, then lift the lid and check on the amount of liquid remaining. If there is still a large amount of liquid, leave the lid off for a further 5 minutes or until the pieces of cauliflower are tender; otherwise replace the lid, but keep checking. After 5 minutes the sauce should be reduced to almost nothing; increase the heat briefly, if necessary, to reduce it further but don't stir the curry too much or the florets may break up.

As soon as the cauliflower is tender and the sauce is much reduced, spoon the curry into serving bowls. Top each helping with a generous spoonful of yoghurt and scatter the top with a few almonds or some coriander leaves. Serve immediately.

Green vegetable gratin
Serves 1

1 medium tomato, chopped
½ medium courgette
 (about 50 g/1¾ oz)
½ tsp olive oil
½ small leek, trimmed
 and chopped
 (about 80 g/2¾ oz)
1 garlic clove, finely
 chopped
50 g(1¾ oz) frozen soya
 beans
several florets of broccoli
(about 80 g/2¾ oz)

30 g (1 oz) Edam cheese,
 grated
black pepper

SERVINGS		NUTRITIONAL INFO	
Protein	1	Calories	262
Fat	0	Carbohydrate	11 g
Dairy	1	Protein	22 g
Fruit	0	Fibre	10 g
Vegetables	4	Salt	0.8 g

Preheat the oven to 180°C/350°F/Gas Mark 4. You will need a small ovenproof dish – it should be about 5 cm (2 in) deep.

Put the chopped tomato in a small non-stick pan with a tablespoon of water. Bring to a simmer and keep an eye on it – there isn't much liquid so you may need to add more water to prevent it from sticking to the bottom of the pan (this will depend on how juicy the tomato is). While the tomato is cooking, chop the courgette across into round slices.

When the tomato is soft, remove from the heat and pour into a sieve over a small bowl, pressing through firmly; discard the pulp.

Rinse the tomato pan, add the olive oil and return the pan to the heat. Add the leek and garlic and stir in the hot oil for a minute or so, until they just begin to take on colour. Then pour the sieved tomato sauce back in the pan and cook it until it has reduced by half, for about a minute. Meanwhile, put a pan of water on to boil. As soon as it is boiling, add the frozen soya beans and cook them for a minute. Then add the broccoli florets and cook for further couple of minutes, and finally add all the courgette rounds and cook everything for a further minute.

Drain the vegetables well. Carefully remove the courgette rounds and set these to one side, then put the rest of the vegetables in the ovenproof dish. Pour over the tomato and leek sauce – don't worry that there doesn't seem to be much – and then place the courgette circles over the top, covering the vegetables. Press the courgettes down gently but firmly. Now scatter the grated Edam over the top, and add plenty of black pepper. Put the dish in the preheated oven and bake for 30 minutes, until the top is golden.

Remove the gratin from the oven and carefully lift the cheesy courgette topping onto one side of a serving plate. Using a slotted spoon, lift the vegetables out and arrange these beside the topping, then spoon a little of the tomato-flavoured liquid on top. Serve immediately.

Tip:

▶ This is a very flexible recipe and invites variations. Still use half a courgette cut into rounds for the topping, and add several good handfuls of dark green kale, roughly chopped. Blanch the kale very briefly in the boiling water just before you drain it.

Refreshing drinks

Ayran yoghurt drink

Serves 1

*100 g (3½ oz) natural
yoghurt
chilled water, still or
sparkling, or soda water*

SERVINGS		NUTRITIONAL INFO	
Protein	0	Calories	79
Fat	0	Carbohydrate	8 g
Dairy	1½	Protein	6 g
Fruit	0	Fibre	0 g
Vegetables	0	Salt	0.2 g

Put the yoghurt in a tall glass and fill the glass with water. Whisk the two together until thoroughly combined and drink immediately.

Green mint tea

Serves 1

You can have unlimited tea. Calorie-free.

*large handful of fresh mint
1 green tea bag*

Strip the leaves from the stems. Warm a teapot, jug or bowl with boiling water, discard it and then add the mint leaves. Add just enough water to cover the leaves, swirl it around the pot and then pour out the water, retaining the leaves. Next add the tea bag and refill the pot with boiling water. Leave for 10 minutes to infuse before drinking.

Lemon and ginger tea

Serves 1

> You can have unlimited tea. Calorie-free.

half lemon
2 cm (½ in) square piece of fresh ginger root, peeled

Cut a slice off the lemon, then squeeze the juice from the rest of the fruit into a heatproof glass or mug. Grate as much of the ginger root as possible into the glass. Top with boiling water, add the slice of lemon, stir well and leave for 5 minutes before drinking.

Tips:

▶ For a savoury drink, dissolve ¼ teaspoon of yeast extract in hot water.

▶ Make lemon balm tea in the same way as the mint tea above, but leave out the tea bag.

▶ Make chilli 'tea' if you're feeling brave or have a cold coming on: add a small amount of chopped chilli to the lemon and ginger drink above, but pass it through a sieve and into a clean glass before drinking.

▶ Make a cool mint tea as above, but leave out the tea bag and add double the amount of mint. Allow it to cool, then add some of it (to taste) to a glass and top up with sparkling water. Add ice cubes.

10

recipes for unrestricted days

Recipes for the five unrestricted days

Sweets and desserts	
Lemon and blueberry yoghurt cake (V)	301
Yoghurt ice cream with raspberries (V)	302
Individual lemon and honey cheesecakes (V)	303
Crunchy blackberry and apple crumble (V)	304
Crêpes (V)	305
Apricot and apple fruit salad (V)	307
Baked nectarines stuffed with nuts (V)	307
Chocolate and orange mousse (V)	308
Prune delight (V)	310
Apple fool with heather honey (V)	311
Hosaf – Turkish dried fruit salad (V)	312

Breakfast

Porridge with dried fruit
Serves 1

2 heaped tbsp porridge oats
(about 40 g/1½ oz)
1 level tsp sultanas
250 ml (8½ fl oz) water
or skimmed or semi-
skimmed milk
2 dried apricots, chopped

SERVINGS		NUTRITIONAL INFO	
If using skimmed milk:			
Carbohydrate	2	Calories	286
Protein	0	Carbohydrate	53 g
Fat	0	Protein	13 g
Dairy	1	Fibre	5 g
Fruit	1	Salt	0.3 g
Vegetables	0		

Put the oats and the sultanas into a small non-stick pan and add the water or milk. Put the pan on a medium heat and bring it to a simmer. Cook for about 10 minutes, stirring frequently to prevent the porridge from sticking.

By now the porridge should be thickening and bubbling well. Stir as it continues to thicken for another few minutes, or until it reaches the consistency you like. Pour into a bowl and scatter the chopped apricots on top. Serve immediately.

Tips:

▶ As an alternative, add 2 chopped almonds to the apricots.

▶ If you prefer your porridge sweeter stir in 1 teaspoon of clear honey.

Classic muesli
Serves 2

80 g (2¾ oz) rolled oats

4 dried apricots, chopped

4 tbsp unsweetened apple juice

1 dessert apple, unpeeled

2 tbsp low-fat natural yoghurt

6 Brazil nuts, chopped

2 tsp clear honey (optional)

SERVINGS		NUTRITIONAL INFO	
Without honey:			
Carbohydrate	2	Calories	283
Protein	0	Carbohydrate	45 g
Fat	1	Protein	8 g
Dairy	½	Fibre	6 g
Fruit	1	Salt	0.1 g
Vegetables	0		

The evening before you want to eat the muesli, put the oats, chopped apricots and apple juice in a bowl. Stir, cover and leave overnight.

The following morning, grate in the apple and stir well. Add the yoghurt to the mixture and stir that in too. Heat a dry frying pan; when hot, add the chopped nuts, stirring them until they begin to colour. Divide the muesli into two serving bowls and scatter over the toasted nuts. Drizzle the honey over these, if you wish.

Soups

Courgette soup with basil and a tomato salsa
Serves 4

2 tsp olive oil

2 medium onions, peeled and chopped

1 kg (2 lb 4 oz) courgettes, trimmed and roughly chopped

4 garlic cloves, crushed
1 litre (1¾ pints) low-salt
vegetable stock
2 medium tomatoes
handful of basil leaves
black pepper

SERVINGS		NUTRITIONAL INFO	
Carbohydrate	0	Calories	146
Protein	0	Carbohydrate	17 g
Fat	0	Protein	9 g
Dairy	½	Fibre	5 g
Fruit	0	Salt	1 g
Vegetables	4		

To serve:
4 tbsp low-fat Greek yoghurt

Put the olive oil in a non-stick pan over a medium heat, and then add the onion. Cook gently, stirring so they don't stick to the bottom of the pan, for about 5 minutes until beginning to soften. Then add the courgettes and garlic and stir these into the softened onions. Cook for a couple of minutes and add the stock, then increase the heat and bring the soup to a simmer. Cook for about 10 minutes, or until the courgettes are soft.

Make the salsa while the soup is cooking. Chop the tomatoes, finely and put them in a small dish or bowl. Tear some of the basil leaves and add to the dish with a good twist of black pepper; stir everything together. Set aside while you finish the soup.

When the soup is ready, remove the pan from the heat and allow it to cool a little. Blend it until smooth, using either a hand-held blender or a liquidiser. If you're using a liquidiser, put it back into the pan and gently reheat the soup. Tear up the remaining basil leaves, add them to the pan then pour into the serving bowls. Divide the tomato salsa between the bowls, scattering it in the middle, and add a swirl of Greek yoghurt to each bowl. Serve immediately.

Tips:

▶ If you like bread with your soup, choose a wholemeal variety instead of white.

▶ This recipe is suitable for making in larger batches and freezing. If freezing, don't add the salsa!

Lentil soup with spinach and a touch of lemon
Serves 4

125 g (4⅓ oz) green lentils
250 g (8⅔ oz) fresh spinach
   leaves
1 tsp olive oil
1 medium onion, chopped
1 garlic clove, finely chopped
1 tsp tomato purée
750–850 ml (1¼–1½ pints)
   low-salt vegetable stock

SERVINGS		NUTRITIONAL INFO	
Carbohydrate	0	Calories	138
Protein	1½	Carbohydrate	20 g
Fat	0	Protein	10 g
Dairy	0	Fibre	6 g
Fruit	0	Salt	1.1 g
Vegetables	1		

juice of half a small lemon
black pepper

Rinse the lentils in a sieve under running water. Put them in a pan, cover with water and cook over a medium heat for 15–20 minutes, or until they begin to soften. Then drain and rinse them once more. Set aside.

Wash the spinach leaves and remove any really stringy stalks; chop the leaves and tender stalks. Heat the olive oil in a saucepan and add the chopped onion. Cook gently for 10 minutes or until the onion is very soft but not burning, then add the garlic. Cook for a further minute, then stir in the lentils.

Add the wet spinach leaves, plus any chopped stalks to the pan; stir these in. Mix the tomato purée with the stock and add enough of the liquid to the pan to cover the spinach leaves and lentils. Cook for 5 minutes, then add the lemon juice and cook for another 5 minutes (the short cooking time should preserve the vivid green colour of the spinach).

Test that the onions and lentils are really soft and remove the pan from the heat. Allow the soup to cool a little and then blend until it is almost smooth using either a hand-held blender or a liquidiser. If you're using a liquidiser, put the soup back into the pan and gently reheat. Taste for seasoning, adding a little black pepper if you wish, and serve.

Tip:

▶ This recipe is suitable for making into larger batches and freezing.

Creamy mushroom soup

Serves 2

2 tsp rapeseed or other vegetable oil
2 medium onions, chopped
600 g (1 lb 4 oz) large flat or field mushrooms
small pinch cayenne pepper
900 ml (1½ pints) low-salt vegetable stock
200 ml (7 fl oz) semi-skimmed or skimmed milk

sprig of thyme or a pinch of dried mixed herbs
black pepper

SERVINGS		NUTRITIONAL INFO	
Carbohydrate	0	Calories	188
Protein	0	Carbohydrate	20 g
Fat	½	Protein	12 g
Dairy	1	Fibre	6 g
Fruit	0	Salt	1.1 g
Vegetables	5		

To serve:
40 g (1½ oz) no- or low-fat Greek yoghurt

Heat the oil in a large pan over a medium heat. Add the onion and cook gently, stirring, for about 5–10 minutes, until soft but not brown. While the onion is cooking, brush any earth from the mushrooms (only peel them if necessary) and trim the ends off the stalks. Chop the mushrooms into chunks.

Add the cayenne pepper to the pan and stir for a few seconds before adding the mushroom pieces. Stir these for a further couple of minutes, being careful not to let them burn. Add the stock and milk. Strip the leaves from the thyme sprig into the pan or stir in the dried mixed herbs. Simmer the soup for about 20 minutes, then check for seasoning and add black pepper to taste.

Allow the soup to cool slightly and blend it roughly using either a hand-held blender or a liquidiser – it shouldn't be too smooth. Add some more water if necessary, then return it to the pan (if using a liquidiser) and reheat. Serve it with two teaspoons of Greek yoghurt swirled into each bowl.

Tips:

▶ For a chunkier soup, blend only half the soup, and then put it into the pan with the unblended half.

▶ For a more intense flavour use a selection of mushrooms, such as chestnut, forestière or porcini.

▶ This recipe is suitable for making in larger batches and freezing.

Roast red pepper soup

Serves 4

4 red peppers
2 tsp olive oil
1 medium onion, chopped
2 garlic cloves, finely chopped
900 ml–1 litre (1½–1¾ pints)
low-salt vegetable stock
1 x 400 g (14 oz) tin of cannellini beans, drained and rinsed

SERVINGS		NUTRITIONAL INFO	
Carbohydrate	0	Calories	147
Protein	1	Carbohydrate	24 g
Fat	0	Protein	7 g
Dairy	0	Fibre	8 g
Fruit	0	Salt	0.9 g
Vegetables	2		

Preheat the grill. Cut the peppers in half and remove the seeds. Put the oil in a small bowl and lightly brush some on the skin side of the peppers. Put the pepper halves on a baking tray, skin side uppermost. Place the tray under the hot grill. Leave the peppers there until the skins begin to blister and turn black – this can take up to 20 minutes, depending on the heat of the grill.

Take the baking tray out and cover the peppers with a tea towel. Leave them for 10 minutes or until they are cool enough to handle, and then gently peel the skin off the flesh. Discard the skins and chop the flesh; set to one side.

Put the remaining olive oil in a large pan. Add the onion and cook gently for 7–8 minutes, then add the garlic and cook for a further 2–3 minutes. Stir the mixture so that it doesn't stick to the bottom of the pan (if it looks like doing so, add a couple of spoonfuls of stock and cook them off). Then add the chopped peppers and the cannellini beans and stir. Add enough stock to cover the peppers and beans, and simmer for 15 minutes, then take the pan off the heat.

Allow the soup to cool a little before blending until mostly smooth, using either a hand-held blender or a liquidiser. If using a liquidiser, return the soup to the pan and reheat gently. Check for seasoning and serve.

Tips:

▶ If you'd like a non-vegetarian soup, add some chopped cooked chicken breast to the peppers and beans after they have cooked in the stock for 10 minutes. And don't blend it – serve it as a chunky soup instead.

▶ This recipe is suitable for making in larger batches and freezing.

Salads and light bites

Horiatiki salata – Greek salad

Serves 2

1 small cos lettuce or
*   2 lettuce hearts*
4 large ripe tomatoes
½ cucumber, about 180g (6 oz)
1 small red onion or 6 spring
*   onions*
1 tbsp olive oil
1 tsp balsamic vinegar
100 g (3½ oz) feta cheese

20 black olives, pitted and sliced
black pepper

SERVINGS		NUTRITIONAL INFO	
Carbohydrate	0	Calories	265
Protein	0	Carbohydrate	13 g
Fat	2	Protein	11 g
Dairy	1½	Fibre	6 g
Fruit	0	Salt	2.1 g
Vegetables	4		

Wash the lettuce leaves, tear them up and divide them between two serving plates or bowls.

Chop the tomatoes and put them in a bowl. Cut the cucumber in half lengthways then chop it up and add to the tomatoes. Then peel the onion, halve it and slice it finely (if using spring onions, chop finely). Add the onion to the bowl.

Put the oil and vinegar into a small screw-top jar (a clean jam jar, for instance). Put the lid on securely, then shake to make a dressing. Pour this dressing over the tomatoes, cucumber and onion, and stir everything to combine.

Remove the feta from its packaging and rinse it under running water, then pat dry with kitchen paper. On a plate, cut the feta into small cubes – some brands will crumble and others will require cutting. Slide the feta into the bowl with the tomatoes. Give this mixture a final, very gentle, stir and spoon it over the salad leaves. Scatter the olives over the salad, add some black pepper and serve.

White bean salad with hard-boiled eggs

Serves 2

2 eggs
½ x 400 g (14 oz) tin haricot
*   or cannellini beans*
½ x 400 g (14 oz) tin black-
*   eyed beans*
1 medium onion, quartered
1 bay leaf
juice of half a lemon
1 tbsp olive oil
3 celery sticks, chopped
large handful of flat-leaf
*   parsley, chopped*

1 small cos lettuce, leaves
*   separated*
black pepper
10 black olives, pitted and
*   halved*

SERVINGS		NUTRITIONAL INFO	
Carbohydrate	0	Calories	326
Protein	3	Carbohydrate	30 g
Fat	1	Protein	19 g
Dairy	0	Fibre	12 g
Fruit	0	Salt	0.5 g
Vegetables	1½		

Put the eggs in a pan of water and bring to the boil. Cook for 10 minutes, then cool rapidly under a cold tap. Put them in a bowl of iced water and set aside in a cool place.

Drain the tins of beans into a large sieve and rinse them thoroughly. Put the rinsed beans in a large pan over a medium to high heat, add the onion and bay leaf and then cover them with fresh water. Bring the beans to a good rolling simmer and cook for 5 minutes, then drain them well.

Allow the beans to cool a little until they are no longer hot, but still warm; remove the bay leaf and the pieces of onion. Discard the bay leaf, but finely slice two of the onion quarters (or use all if you wish) and put them back into the beans.

In a large bowl mix together the lemon juice, olive oil and chopped celery and parsley. Then add the warm beans and onion, and stir everything well. Cover the beans and leave them to absorb the flavours for 30 minutes.

Wash the lettuce leaves, tear them up and divide between two serving plates. Check the flavour of the beans and add black pepper to taste, then stir once more before dividing between the two plates. Peel the hard-boiled eggs and cut these into quarters. Decorate the salad with the eggs and the olives and serve.

A pair of potato salads
Serves 2

250 g (8⅔ oz) new potatoes, in their skins
2 tsp balsamic vinegar
black pepper
100 g (3½ oz) low-fat natural yoghurt
2 tsp Dijon mustard

Non-vegetarian salad:

1 small red onion, sliced into
   rings
200 g (7 oz) smoked mackerel
squeeze of lemon juice
½–1 tsp horseradish sauce
   (to taste and optional)

SERVINGS		NUTRITIONAL INFO	
Carbohydrate	1	Calories	501
Protein	3½	Carbohydrate	28 g
Fat	0	Protein	25 g
Dairy	½	Fibre	3 g
Fruit	0	Salt	2.7 g
Vegetables	½		

Vegetarian salad:

6 spring onions, chopped
1 ripe avocado, halved and
   stone removed
¼ cucumber, deseeded and
   finely chopped
2 hard-boiled eggs

SERVINGS		NUTRITIONAL INFO	
Carbohydrate	1	Calories	371
Protein	1	Carbohydrate	29 g
Fat	2	Protein	15 g
Dairy	½	Fibre	7 g
Fruit	0	Salt	1 g
Vegetables	1½		

To serve:

black pepper
handful of salad leaves, about 30 g (1 oz)

Chop the new potatoes into pieces no larger than 1.5 cm (½ in) and put them in a pan of cold water. Bring the pan to the boil, cover and cook the potatoes until they are just soft. Drain and put them in a bowl with the balsamic vinegar and some black pepper. Turn the potatoes over carefully with a wooden spoon, then add the yoghurt and mustard and stir the potatoes once more. They should still be quite warm and will absorb the flavours much better than if they were cold.

For the non-vegetarian version, add the red onion to the potatoes and stir it in. Carefully shred the smoked mackerel into medium-sized pieces, removing any bones and skin, and squeeze over a little lemon juice. Put this in with the warm potatoes and the horseradish, if using, and mix everything together well.

For the vegetarian version, add the spring onions to the potatoes. Slice through the flesh of the avocado lengthways and across, just to the skin, but not through it, and then bend the avocado back in on itself. The chunks will either pop out by themselves or will be easy to remove. Add them to the potatoes along with the cucumber, and very gently mix them in. Put some salad leaves on serving plates, and divide the salad between them. Peel the hard-boiled eggs and chop them finely, then scatter over the top of the salad.

Check the seasoning, whichever version, and serve on top of salad leaves (the smoked mackerel salad is particularly good slightly warm).

Warm beetroot and feta salad

Serves 2

10–12 small to medium beetroot, uncooked (about 150 g/5 oz)

1 bag of mixed salad leaves, about 120 g (4 oz)

100 g (3½ oz) feta cheese

1 small red onion, finely sliced

1 tsp olive oil

1 tsp lemon juice

leaves from small sprig of thyme

black pepper

SERVINGS		NUTRITIONAL INFO	
Carbohydrate	0	Calories	204
Protein	0	Carbohydrate	12 g
Fat	½	Protein	10 g
Dairy	1½	Fibre	4 g
Fruit	0	Salt	2 g
Vegetables	2		

Preheat the oven to 200°C/400°F/Gas Mark 6. Gently clean the raw beetroot but don't scrub, peel or top and tail them;

just trim off the leaves, leaving about 1 cm (¼ in) of stalk. Tear off a large piece of foil and put the beetroot on it, then seal the foil over to form a flat parcel. Put the parcel on a baking tray and bake in the oven until the beetroot give slightly when you squeeze the parcel; they will take at least 30 minutes, but the cooking time will depend on their size. Test that they are cooked by unwrapping the parcel and sticking a knife in one – it should go in gently, and the skin should also be a little wrinkled.

Carefully unwrap the parcel and allow the beetroot to cool until they can just be handled. Then slide off the skins; these should come away easily, but may need encouragement with a knife. Put the peeled beetroot to one side. (If using cooked beetroot, see tip below; clean them if necessary and pop them in a preheated oven for 5 minutes to warm up – they just need to be warm, not recooked.)

Divide the salad leaves between two plates. Chop the warm beetroot and scatter the pieces over the leaves. Then rinse the feta cheese, pat dry on kitchen paper and crumble it evenly over the beetroot. Scatter the red onion on top, to taste. Make a dressing by whisking together the olive oil, lemon juice and thyme leaves in a small bowl, and pour it over the salad. Add some black pepper and serve immediately.

Tip:

▶ If it is impossible to find raw beetroot, use cooked ones – just omit the roasting instructions; instead, warm briefly as instructed in the method above. If the only raw beetroot you can find are enormous, then definitely use smaller cooked ones. The only beets to avoid are those pickled in vinegar!

Tuna and mixed bean salad
Serves 2

1 x 400 g (14 oz) tin of mixed beans (pulses) in water

1 garlic clove, peeled but whole

1 tbsp olive oil

1 tsp balsamic vinegar

½ tsp Dijon mustard

squeeze of lemon juice

10 spring onions, finely sliced

5 radishes, trimmed, halved and finely sliced

small handful of flat-leaf parsley (optional), finely chopped

1 x 160–185 g (5½–6½ oz) tin tuna steak in spring water

black pepper

1 packet rocket or similarly strong-tasting salad leaves, about 140 g (5 oz)

SERVINGS		NUTRITIONAL INFO	
Carbohydrate	0	Calories	281
Protein	4	Carbohydrate	25 g
Fat	1	Protein	26 g
Dairy	0	Fibre	11 g
Fruit	0	Salt	0.4 g
Vegetables	1½		

Drain and rinse the mixed beans and put them in a pan with the garlic. Cover with fresh water, put the pan over a medium to high heat and bring the beans to a simmer. Turn the heat off and cover the pan; set aside for a couple of minutes while making the dressing.

Put the olive oil, vinegar and mustard in a small bowl and squeeze in some lemon juice. Then whisk well to combine all the ingredients into a vinaigrette dressing. Drain the warm beans, remove the garlic clove, and put the beans in a large bowl. Pour the dressing over them and stir well. Set aside for 10 minutes or so to cool down.

Add the sliced spring onions and radishes to the beans, then the parsley (if using) and stir everything together.

Drain the tuna and flake the fish onto the beans, keeping the flakes as large as possible. Add some black pepper and then carefully mix the tuna and the beans together, trying not to break up the tuna too much. Divide the salad leaves between two plates and spoon the tuna and bean salad on top. Serve immediately.

Tip:

▶ This recipe requires a tin of mixed pulses – generally including chickpeas, borlotti, kidney and haricot beans, however don't use the ones containing green beans!

Tabbouleh
Serves 4

100 g (3½ oz) couscous or bulgur wheat
juice of 1 large lemon
2 large bunches of flat-leaf parsley, about 200 g (7 oz)
small bunch of fresh mint
3 large tomatoes, finely chopped
2 medium red onions, finely chopped
1 tbsp olive oil
black pepper

SERVINGS		NUTRITIONAL INFO	
Carbohydrate	1	Calories	140
Protein	0	Carbohydrate	24 g
Fat	½	Protein	5 g
Dairy	0	Fibre	5 g
Fruit	0	Salt	<0.1 g
Vegetables	2		

Put the couscous or bulgur wheat in a bowl and cover it well with boiling water (or follow the instructions on the packet). Stir well, then cover the bowl and set it to one side for about 5 minutes; then stir it again, breaking up any lumps. Test a few grains – they should be soft – but leave for another few minutes if they are not. Drain off any excess water in a sieve and squeeze the grains dry by pressing with the back of a wooden spoon. Rinse out the empty bowl and dry it off, then pour in the lemon juice. Put the warm grains back in the bowl and stir it well to incorporate the lemon juice.

Discard the tough stalks of the parsley and mint (cut these off while the herbs are still in bunches). Finely chop the leaves and put in a large bowl, then add the chopped tomatoes and onion. Tip in the couscous or bulgur wheat and add the olive oil and some black pepper. Combine everything together thoroughly, check the seasoning and serve.

Tips:

▶ This refreshing Mediterranean salad should be made with lots of parsley, and it's delicious as an accompaniment to cold chicken, such as 'Baked chicken with rosemary' (see page 276).

▶ If available, choose wholewheat couscous over ordinary couscous; just follow the instructions on the packet.

Red cabbage coleslaw with nuts and seeds
Serves 2

100 g (3½ oz) red cabbage
2 medium carrots, peeled
1 large celery stick (optional)
1 medium red onion
3 tbsp low-fat mayonnaise
4 walnut halves, chopped
2 tsp pumpkin seeds
black pepper

SERVINGS		NUTRITIONAL INFO	
Carbohydrate	0	Calories	194
Protein	0	Carbohydrate	15 g
Fat	2	Protein	4 g
Dairy	0	Fibre	6 g
Fruit	0	Salt	0.7 g
Vegetables	2½		

Using a large knife, finely shred the cabbage and put it in a large mixing bowl. Grate the carrots using a coarse grater and put them in the bowl, too. Pull the strings off the outside of the celery, slice it lengthways and then finely chop. Next slice the onion into rings and cut these into sections. Add the chopped celery and onions to the bowl and give everything a good stir, mixing it well.

Add the mayonnaise and a good grind of black pepper to the bowl, and then stir again to mix the mayonnaise with all the vegetables. If you are serving the coleslaw immediately, chop the walnuts and scatter these over the coleslaw with the pumpkin seeds. If you plan to serve the salad later, cover the coleslaw and refrigerate it, then add the nuts and seeds just before serving.

Tips:

▶ This healthy coleslaw is good by itself, or perhaps with a wholemeal crusty roll or oat cakes. It's also delicious with cold chicken and makes a great packed lunch.

▶ When red cabbage isn't available, just use white cabbage.

Fish and seafood

Prawns with beans, tomatoes and thyme
Serves 2

1 x 400 g (14 oz) tin borlotti
  beans
250 g (8 ⅔ oz) fresh tomatoes
200 g (7 oz) raw prawns
2 tsp olive oil
1 garlic clove, finely chopped
1 sprig thyme
black pepper

SERVINGS		NUTRITIONAL INFO	
Carbohydrate	0	Calories	241
Protein	4	Carbohydrate	25 g
Fat	½	Protein	27 g
Dairy	0	Fibre	9 g
Fruit	0	Salt	0.6 g
Vegetables	1½		

Drain and rinse the beans. Chop the tomatoes roughly and rinse the prawns under a cold tap.

Put the olive oil in a non-stick frying pan over a medium heat. When it is warm, add the tomatoes and the garlic and cook them together for a couple of minutes. Strip the leaves off the thyme and add them to the pan, and then add the beans. Add the prawns and cook for about 5 minutes until they turn pink and are cooked through. During this time add a little water to keep the mixture from sticking to the bottom of the pan; a couple of tablespoons should be enough – the dish should be lightly sauced – but this will depend on how juicy the tomatoes were. Check for seasoning and add black pepper to taste. Serve immediately, perhaps with wholemeal or crusty granary bread to mop up the sauce.

Tip:

▶ If you cannot buy raw prawns you can use cooked prawns

instead but this will increase the salt content. Cooked prawns should only be gently warmed to avoid overcooking. Add after you have cooked the beans for about 5 minutes.

Quick fish curry

Serves 4

750 g (1 lb 9 oz) cod loin

2 tsp rapeseed or other
    neutral-tasting oil

2 medium onions, finely
    chopped

2 garlic cloves, finely
    chopped

2 tsp garam masala

½ tsp cayenne pepper

½ tsp turmeric

black pepper

1 tbsp tomato purée

350 ml (12 fl oz) water

squeeze of lemon juice

SERVINGS		NUTRITIONAL INFO	
with rice:			
Carbohydrate	2	Calories	415
Protein	3	Carbohydrate	56 g
Fat	0	Protein	40 g
Dairy	0	Fibre	4 g
Fruit	0	Salt	0.3 g
Vegetables	½		

To serve:

240 g (8 oz) basmati rice,
    brown if possible

The rice will probably take longer than the curry (depending on the brand and whether it is brown or white), so prepare it according to the instructions on the packet before starting the curry itself.

Carefully remove the skin from the fish and discard any bones you come across, then cut the fish into pieces no smaller than about 3 cm (1 in) square. Heat the oil in a pan or heat-proof casserole over a medium heat and add the onion and garlic. Cook these for about 5 minutes, or until the onion begins to soften but has not begun to take on much colour.

Add the garam masala, cayenne pepper, turmeric and some black pepper and stir, then add the tomato purée. Stir once, then quickly add the water and let the sauce come to a steady but gentle simmer. Carefully add the pieces of fish and cover the pan.

Cook the curry for 10 minutes, then lift the lid and check that the fish is cooking well. If the sauce is nicely reduced, put the lid back on and cook the curry for another 5 minutes; if there is still plenty of sauce, leave the lid off to reduce it further, but be careful the curry doesn't stick to the bottom of the pan. It is important not to stir the curry too much or the pieces of fish will break up. Just before serving, add a squeeze of lemon juice and a little pepper (taste before seasoning), stir carefully; serve the curry with the rice.

Tip:

▶ This delicious fish curry could be served with steamed spinach.

Kedgeree with fresh salmon
Serves 2

2 small salmon fillets, skin removed, about 100 g (3½ oz) each
1 large egg, hard-boiled
60 g (2 oz) basmati rice, preferably brown
1 tsp rapeseed oil
1 medium onion, peeled and chopped

SERVINGS		NUTRITIONAL INFO	
Using brown basmati rice:			
Carbohydrate	1	Calories	388
Protein	4	Carbohydrate	31 g
Fat	0	Protein	28 g
Dairy	0	Fibre	3 g
Fruit	0	Salt	0.3 g
Vegetables	½		

*1 garlic clove, finely chopped
(optional)
½ tsp garam masala or mild
curry powder*

*handful of flat-leaf parsley,
chopped*

Put the salmon in a microwaveable dish. Cover it with cling-film, puncture the film in several places and microwave at full power for 1½ minutes. Check to see that the fish flakes easily, and set it aside if it does so (if not, give it another 30 seconds, continuing until it is ready). If you haven't got a microwave, put the salmon fillets in a pan and add enough water to come halfway up the sides. Poach over a medium heat until the fish flakes easily, which will probably take less than 10 minutes, depending on the thickness of the fillets. Flake the fish and set it to one side. Hard-boil the egg, rinse under cold water and leave it in cold water to cool down.

Rinse the rice under running water and put it in a non- stick pan. Cover the rice with water and bring to the boil. Lower the heat until the rice is simmering, then cover the pan and cook the rice until most of the water has been absorbed and the rice is tender (check that it isn't sticking). This will take 15–25 minutes depending on whether you use white or brown rice.

While the rice is cooking, peel the hard-boiled egg and cut it into quarters. Heat the oil in a large non-stick frying pan. Cook the chopped onion very gently until it has softened, and then add the garlic (if using) and garam masala. Stir to combine.

Drain the rice and add it to the pan; stir it well in order to blend everything together. Then carefully add the flaked fish and stir it, very gently this time, until thoroughly mixed. Make sure the salmon is warmed through then divide the kedgeree between the serving dishes. Garnish each serving with pieces of hard-boiled egg and a scatter of chopped parsley, and serve immediately.

Tip:

▶ Kedgeree is often used as a brunch dish, but it makes a great choice for supper, too. For supper, serve it with steamed vegetables or a couple of salads – a plain green salad and one featuring tomatoes and spring onions would be especially good.

Salmon with lentils
Serves 2

100 g (3½ oz) Puy lentils (uncooked weight)
1 small onion, peeled and halved
1 garlic clove, peeled but whole
1 bay leaf
1 sprig of thyme
½ tsp olive oil
1 tbsp low-fat cream cheese
black pepper

2 salmon fillets, skin removed, approximately 120 g (4 oz) each

SERVINGS		NUTRITIONAL INFO	
Carbohydrate	0	Calories	404
Protein	6	Carbohydrate	28 g
Fat	0	Protein	39 g
Dairy	½	Fibre	7 g
Fruit	0	Salt	0.3 g
Vegetables	½		

Rinse the lentils, then put them in a pan with half of the onion, the garlic clove, bay leaf and sprig of thyme. Cover with water and bring to the boil. Reduce the heat to a simmer and cook until the lentils are tender but not soft or mushy. This shouldn't take longer than 30 minutes. Drain the lentils and discard the half onion, garlic, bay leaf and the stalk of the thyme – most of the leaves will have come off.

Finely chop the remaining half onion. Put the oil in a pan over a medium heat and fry the onion gently for 3–4 minutes. Add the lentils and heat through, then take off the heat and allow to cool for two or three minutes before stirring in the cream cheese. Season with black pepper and cover the pan to keep the lentils warm while you cook the salmon.

Heat a non-stick frying pan over a medium to high heat. Place the salmon fillets in the pan and cook them gently on one side for about 2 minutes until they just begin to colour. Then turn them over and cook the other side, also for about 2 minutes. Check the salmon is cooked right through (this will depend on the thickness of the fillets), and take the pan off the heat.

Divide the lentils between two warmed plates. Gently place a fillet of salmon on top, and serve immediately.

Tip:

▶ Puy lentils are readily available and don't need preliminary soaking. They also have a lovely nutty taste and are really nutritious.

Fish couscous
Serves 4

500 g (1 lb 1 oz) firm white fish (cod loin, haddock, monkfish tail)
1 x 400 g (14 oz) tin chickpeas
2 tsp olive oil
2 medium onions, finely chopped

SERVINGS		NUTRITIONAL INFO	
Carbohydrate	2	Calories	359
Protein	3	Carbohydrate	48 g
Fat	0	Protein	33 g
Dairy	0	Fibre	9 g
Fruit	0	Salt	0.3 g
Vegetables	2		

2 garlic cloves, chopped
1 tsp ground cumin
½ tsp cayenne pepper
½ tsp ras el hanout (or
*   'Tunisian spice blend'),*
*   optional*
2 medium carrots, peeled
*   and chopped*

1 medium red pepper,
*   deseeded and chopped*
1 medium yellow pepper,
*   deseeded and chopped*
4 tsp tomato purée dissolved
*   in 400 ml (14 fl oz) hot*
*   water*
175 g (6 oz) couscous

Cut the fish into large pieces, put them in a bowl, cover and put in the refrigerator. If you are using monkfish you may need to fillet it first. Slice the fillets away from the central bone with a really sharp knife, then cut away the membrane on the outside. Discard the bone and membrane and chop the flesh. Drain and rinse the chickpeas thoroughly.

Put the oil in a large pan over a medium heat. Add the onions and cook them, stirring, for 5 minutes. Then add the garlic and stir in the spices, and cook for a further minute, still stirring well. Add the carrot and peppers to the pan, mixing them in, then add the tomato purée diluted in water. Simmer for 15 minutes, then add the chickpeas and the fish. Add enough water, if necessary, to cover everything – this fish stew should be quite liquid. Partly cover the pan and cook for a further 6–10 minutes, depending on the type of fish used. The vegetables and the fish should be cooked but not breaking up, the chickpeas should be really soft and the liquid will have reduced a little.

Towards the end of cooking, prepare the couscous. Either follow the instructions on the packet or put the dried couscous in a large bowl and pour over boiling water to cover it well. Stir with a fork, cover the bowl and wait until the grains have absorbed most of the water, which will only take a few minutes. Stir a couple of times, then drain the couscous well through a fine sieve.

Put a serving of couscous on each plate and ladle the fish, vegetables and sauce over it. Serve immediately.

Tip:

▶ If available, choose wholewheat couscous. This recipe also works well with bulgur wheat.

Smoked fishcakes
Serves 4 (makes 8 fishcakes)

600 g (1 lb 4 oz) smoked haddock fillets, skin removed, undyed if possible
400 g (14 oz) new potatoes in their skins, chopped
black pepper
8 spring onions, trimmed and finely chopped
1 egg, beaten
1 tbsp wholemeal flour

SERVINGS		NUTRITIONAL INFO	
Carbohydrate	1½	Calories	319
Protein	2½	Carbohydrate	30 g
Fat	1	Protein	35 g
Dairy	0	Fibre	3 g
Fruit	0	Salt	3.2 g
Vegetables	0		

2 tbsp wholemeal breadcrumbs
2 tbsp rapeseed or other neutral-tasting oil
1 lemon, quartered

Cook the fish, either in a microwave or a pan. To microwave, put the fillets in a microwave-proof dish, add a couple of tablespoons of water, cover with clingfilm and pierce the film in several places with a knife. Then microwave on full power until the fish is cooked and the flesh flakes easily; this should take about 2–3 minutes at 800W. Once the fish is done, lift it out of the dish and put on a plate, but keep the cooking liquid. If cooking the fish on the hob, put the fillets in a large pan over a medium heat, cover with water and poach until done – again, save the cooking liquid. This takes about 5 minutes depending on the thickness of the fillet.

Boil the potatoes until soft then drain. Add some black pepper and a little of the fish-cooking liquid – they should be quite dry – and mash them until they are smooth, then transfer to a bowl. Flake the fish well and add it to the pota- toes, then add the spring onions. Add about two-thirds of the beaten egg and stir everything together with a wooden spoon. Then cover the bowl and put it in the refrigerator for 30 minutes or so.

Cover a large baking tray (or two smaller ones) with grease- proof paper or foil. Dust the flour onto a board or work surface, put the rest of the beaten egg in a bowl and the breadcrumbs on a plate. Take the fishcake mixture out of the refrigerator and, using a spoon, divide the mix into eight. One at a time, rub your hands with the flour and roll each serving between your hands into a ball, then press it gently into a fat fishcake shape. Dip each cake briefly in the reserved beaten egg, then roll in the breadcrumbs, covering all the surfaces. Put the finished fishcakes on the baking tray. When they are all done, put the tray in the refrigerator for 20–30 minutes to chill.

Put the oil in a large non-stick frying pan over a medium heat. Once it is hot, carefully lift the fishcakes in and cook them gently, turning them over to do each side – how long this takes will depend on how fat they are, but it shouldn't be more than about 8 minutes. Drain them on kitchen paper and then serve immediately with the lemon quarters and perhaps with steamed spinach or a rocket and tomato salad on the side.

Caribbean prawns and rice
Serves 2

1 medium tomato

100 g (3½ oz) long-grain
  brown rice

1 tsp olive oil

1 small onion, peeled and
  finely chopped

2 garlic cloves, crushed

1 red pepper, deseeded and
  chopped

1 chilli, deseeded and finely
  chopped or a pinch of
  cayenne pepper

500 ml (17 fl oz) low-salt
  vegetable stock

½ tsp paprika

300 g (10½ oz) raw king
  prawns

handful of coriander leaves,
  chopped (optional)

SERVINGS		NUTRITIONAL INFO	
Carbohydrate	1½	Calories	405
Protein	3	Carbohydrate	59 g
Fat	0	Protein	33 g
Dairy	0	Fibre	5 g
Fruit	0	Salt	1.6 g
Vegetables	2		

Chop the tomato and put it to one side. Rinse the rice under a running tap.

Put the oil in a large frying pan with a lid (an ordinary pan will do if necessary) and warm it over a medium heat. Add the onion, garlic, red pepper and the chilli, if using, and fry them gently until they soften and begin to change colour. Then add the stock, the chopped tomato, the pinch of cayenne (if using instead of chilli) and the paprika. Bring the liquid to a simmer and cover the pan.

Add the rice, then simmer on a low heat until it is tender and almost all the liquid has been absorbed – the time will vary so check regularly, but it will probably be about 25 minutes. If the rice shows signs of drying out completely, add a little boiling water; if there seems to be a lot of liquid, increase the temperature slightly to cook it off. As soon as the rice is ready, add the prawns and cook until pink and cooked through. Take the pan off the heat and serve immediately, with the coriander leaves scattered on top.

Tips:

▶ Make this dish as hot as you like – just add more chilli.

▶ Sliced avocado and a celery salad would make excellent accompaniments.

▶ If you cannot buy raw prawns you can use cooked prawns instead but they are higher in salt. Cooked prawns should only be gently warmed to avoid overcooking.

Chicken

Baked chicken with rosemary

Serves 2

2 skinless chicken breasts, about 125 g (4 oz) each
1 tsp olive oil
3 sprigs of rosemary
2 garlic cloves, cut into quarters
juice of 1 lemon

SERVINGS		NUTRITIONAL INFO	
Carbohydrate	0	Calories	159
Protein	4	Carbohydrate	1 g
Fat	0	Protein	28 g
Dairy	0	Fibre	<1 g
Fruit	0	Salt	0.3 g
Vegetables	0		

Preheat the oven to 200°C/400°F/Gas Mark 6. Remove the skin from the chicken breasts (if not skinless) and discard it.

Drizzle the oil into an ovenproof dish, swirl it around and put the dish in the oven until the oil is hot. Take the dish out of the oven and turn the chicken breasts in the oil to seal them and brown them slightly, then take them out and put them on a plate.

Put the whole sprigs of rosemary in the dish, then scatter in the pieces of garlic. Put the chicken breasts on top of the rosemary, right side up. Make the lemon juice up to 100 ml (3½ fl oz) with water and pour it over the chicken.

Return the dish to the oven and cook the chicken for 20 minutes. Then turn the breasts over, cook for a further 5–10 minutes before turning them the right way up again and cooking until they are done: the juice should run clear when you stick a knife into the thickest part. This will probably take another 10 minutes, depending on the size of the chicken breasts. Once the chicken is ready, lift it out of the dish and allow any excess lemony liquid to run off before serving. Serve the breasts immediately, or chill them thoroughly once they have cooled down.

Tips:

▶ These chicken breasts are ideal hot or cold with steamed vegetables, a tomato salad or a baked potato.

▶ Pasta makes a good accompaniment when they're hot, especially if you spoon some of the lemony liquid over the pasta before serving.

▶ Cold and sliced, these are great as a sandwich ingredient or part of a salad.

Mediterranean chicken casserole
Serves 4

3 medium onions, peeled

1 tbsp olive oil

4 chicken breasts, skin removed, about 125 g (4 ⅓ oz) each

1 large green pepper, deseeded and chopped

2 garlic cloves, peeled and finely chopped

1 x 400 g (14 oz) tin chopped tomatoes

2 sprigs of thyme, leaves stripped

1 sprig of fresh oregano or marjoram (if available), leaves stripped

100 ml (3½ fl oz) chicken or vegetable stock

15 black olives, pitted and halved

SERVINGS		NUTRITIONAL INFO	
Carbohydrate	0	Calories	233
Protein	4	Carbohydrate	14 g
Fat	1	Protein	31 g
Dairy	0	Fibre	4 g
Fruit	0	Salt	0.9 g
Vegetables	1½		

Slice one of the onions into rings and finely chop the other two. Heat the olive oil in a large pan or heatproof casserole over a medium to high heat. Cut the chicken breasts into pieces no larger than 1.5 cm (½ in) square, and add them to the pan once the oil is hot. You may need to do this in several batches to prevent overcrowding. Stir the pieces round, sealing and browning them slightly, and then lift them out of the pan and put aside.

Lower the heat and add the onions, green pepper and garlic. Cook gently in what remains of the oil, until they are beginning to soften and brown, and stirring so they do not stick to the bottom of the pan. Then return the chicken pieces to the pan and pour in the chopped tomatoes. Add the stripped leaves from the thyme and marjoram or oregano. Finally, add the stock, bring up to a simmer, then cover the pan and cook gently for about 30–35 minutes. Check it and give it a stir halfway through the cooking time.

After 35 minutes, add the olives and check the level of liquid. The final sauce should be thick, so if it looks a little thin, raise the heat and take off the lid. Cook for another 10 minutes, or until the chicken is really tender and the vegetables are soft and melting. Check for seasoning, stir gently, and serve.

Tips:

▶ This chicken dish is lovely by itself with steamed vegetables or a green salad, but it is also good with boiled rice or new potatoes.

▶ A pinch of dried mixed herbs – herbes de Provence or an Italian blend – can be used instead of the fresh thyme and marjoram.

▶ This recipe freezes very well.

Chicken tagine with carrots and chickpeas
Serves 4

425 g (15 oz) chicken breasts, skin removed

2 tsp olive oil

1 medium onion, roughly chopped

3 medium carrots, chopped

¼ tsp ground ginger

¼ tsp cinnamon

SERVINGS		NUTRITIONAL INFO	
Carbohydrate	½	Calories	217
Protein	4	Carbohydrate	16 g
Fat	0	Protein	27 g
Dairy	0	Fibre	5 g
Fruit	0	Salt	0.3 g
Vegetables	1		

juice of half a lemon
1 x 210 g (7½ oz) can
   chickpeas, drained and
   rinsed

2 tsp tomato purée
400–500 ml (14–17 fl oz)
   water or chicken stock
2 tsp honey

Cut the chicken breasts into pieces no bigger than 2 cm (½ in) square. Heat the oil in a large heavy-bottomed saucepan or heatproof casserole over a medium heat. Add the chopped onion and carrots and cook gently until the onion just begins to change colour.

Add the chicken pieces and stir for a minute or so. Keep stir- ring to make sure the chicken pieces don't stick to the bottom of the pan, and then add the spices and the lemon juice. Stir everything well to coat the chicken in the spices, then add the chickpeas, tomato purée and enough stock or water to cover the chicken.

Cook for 30 minutes, uncovered, then add the honey. Continue cooking for a further 10 minutes or until the sauce is much reduced. If you're intending to serve the tagine with couscous or bulgur wheat, don't reduce the sauce too much.

Tip:
▶ Instead of the carrots, substitute half a small butternut squash, peeled, deseeded and chopped.

Chicken fajitas
Serves 4

500 g (1 lb 1 oz) skinless
   chicken breasts
2 limes

½ tsp paprika
1 tsp ground cumin

1 red chilli, deseeded and
   finely chopped, or ½ tsp
   chilli powder
black pepper
2 tsp olive oil
1 red pepper, deseeded and
   finely chopped
1 green pepper, deseeded and
   finely chopped
1 medium red onion
1 tsp tomato purée

SERVINGS		NUTRITIONAL INFO	
Carbohydrate	2	Calories	381
Protein	4	Carbohydrate	49 g
Fat	0	Protein	36 g
Dairy	½	Fibre	5 g
Fruit	0	Salt	0.8 g
Vegetables	2		

To serve:
salad leaves
bunch of coriander, leaves only

150 g (5 oz) low-fat natural
   yoghurt
4 tortilla wraps

Cut the chicken breast into fine strips, no longer than 3.5 cm
(1½ in) and no larger than 1 cm (¼ in) deep and wide. Squeeze
one of the limes into a large mixing bowl and add the paprika,
cumin, chilli or chilli powder and a good grinding of black
pepper. Add a teaspoon of olive oil as well, then stir everything
together. Add the chicken and mix it in with a wooden spoon.
Set the bowl to one side.

In the meantime, prepare the peppers, cut the onion in half
and then into slices. Add the vegetables to the chicken bowl,
together with the juice of the other lime, and stir well.

Put some crisp salad leaves on each serving plate, and remove
the leaves from the coriander. Pour the yoghurt into a small bowl.
If you want to heat the tortillas in the oven, preheat it and put them
in (following the instructions on the packet), or use a microwave.

Warm a large non-stick frying pan or wok on a high heat and
add a teaspoon of oil. When smoking, tip in the chicken mixture

Cook, stirring constantly to prevent it burning, for 5 minutes. Then add the tomato purée and stir it in. Continue cooking and stirring for a further minute or until you are sure the chicken is cooked – it should be beginning to crisp a little at the edges and will be opaque all the way through. Remove from the heat.

Then assemble the fajitas: spoon some yoghurt on each tortilla wrap, scatter some coriander leaves over it, and divide the chicken between them. Add a little more yoghurt and then wrap the tortilla over. Serve immediately.

Tip:

▶ You can also use turkey breast or steak in this recipe instead of the chicken, and include some guacamole (see page 195) when you wrap the fajitas.

Meat

Homemade classic burgers
Serves 4 (makes 4 burgers)

500 g (1 lb 1 oz) lean beef
 mince
black pepper
1 large sprig of thyme, leaves
 stripped
2 tsp Dijon or wholegrain
 mustard (optional)
2 small egg yolks, or
1 large one

SERVINGS		NUTRITIONAL INFO	
Carbohydrate	0	Calories	254
Protein	4	Carbohydrate	<1 g
Fat	0	Protein	29 g
Dairy	0	Fibre	0 g
Fruit	0	Salt	0.6 g
Vegetables	0		

Put the beef in a bowl, grind some black pepper over it and mix it well with a wooden spoon, breaking up any chunks. Then add the leaves from the thyme, the mustard and the egg yolks and combine. The mixture will come together, but do not overwork the meat as it will toughen the burgers. Divide it into four equal amounts and form into four patties.

Heat the grill to a high temperature. Put a large piece of foil on the grill pan then carefully lift the patties onto the foil with a spatula. Cook them under the grill for 5–10 minutes, turning once until they are done to your satisfaction. How long this takes will depend on how thick they are as well as how you like them done – rare, medium or well done. Serve immediately.

Vegetarian alternative:

Drain and rinse two 400 g (14 oz) tins of kidney beans in water. Put them in a pan, cover with fresh water and bring to the boil, then drain the beans again (this makes them easier to mash), and put them in a bowl. Add 100g (3½ oz) wholemeal breadcrumbs and mash together with the beans, then add the thyme, mustard and egg yolks and stir everything thoroughly. Form into 4 patties, as above, then put them on a baking tray and grill for 5–6 minutes on each side.

SERVINGS		NUTRITIONAL INFO	
Carbohydrate	1	Calories	248
Protein	2	Carbohydrate	41 g
Fat	0	Protein	15 g
Dairy	0	Fibre	10 g
Fruit	0	Salt	0.8 g
Vegetables	0		

Tips:

▶ These burgers are simple, healthy and quick to make and you can vary the flavourings to suit your personal taste. Try adding some ground cumin, finely chopped chilli and maybe coriander leaves for a hot and spicy burger, or add a bit of cinnamon and cumin for a North African tang.

▶ Baked potatoes and a tomato salad would make a great accompaniment.

Marinated lamb and red onion kebabs with a yoghurt and herb sauce
Serves 2

250 g (8⅔ oz) lean lamb
   steaks
3 tbsp low-fat natural
   yoghurt
1 tsp olive oil
1 bay leaf black pepper
1 medium red onion

SERVINGS		NUTRITIONAL INFO	
Carbohydrate	0	Calories	374
Protein	4	Carbohydrate	22 g
Fat	0	Protein	36 g
Dairy	1½	Fibre	2 g
Fruit	0	Salt	0.6 g
Vegetables	½		

For the sauce:
250 g (8⅔ oz) low- or no-fat
   Greek yoghurt
large handful of mint leaves,
   finely chopped
pinch paprika

To serve:
handful of coriander leaves

NB: The lamb needs to marinate for several hours or overnight – if it goes into its marinade and into the refrigerator at the start of the day it will be ready to cook that night.

Cut the lamb steaks into 1.5 cm (½ in) cubes, and discard any fat that is easily detached. Put the lamb cubes into a bowl and spoon the 3 tablespoons of yoghurt and oil over them.

Add the bay leaf and turn the meat over in the yoghurt until thoroughly coated. Grind over a little black pepper, cover the bowl with clingfilm and put it in the refrigerator to marinate.

If you intend to use bamboo skewers for the kebabs, soak them in water for half an hour before you cook. Make the yoghurt and herb sauce by putting the Greek yoghurt and chopped mint leaves into a bowl. Stir, then sprinkle a little paprika over the top. Pop the dressing in the refrigerator while you prepare and cook the kebabs.

Preheat the grill to a high temperature. Cut the red onion into quarters, then separate each quarter into individual pieces, and take the meat out of the refrigerator. Thread pieces of onion on to the skewers alternately with cubes of meat, then rest the ends of the completed skewers over a roasting tin or baking tray so that the meat is suspended above it.

Put the kebabs under the grill and cook, turning them a couple of times until they are done to your taste – this will probably take about 10–15 minutes. Serve immediately with a dollop of the yoghurt sauce and a scatter of coriander leaves.

Thai-style stir-fried beef with lime, red onion and cucumber

Serves 2

240 g (8 oz) stir-fry beef or
  beef sirloin
1 lemon grass stick
2 limes
1 red chilli (or to taste)
½ cucumber

SERVINGS		NUTRITIONAL INFO	
Carbohydrate	2	Calories	447
Protein	4	Carbohydrate	57 g
Fat	½	Protein	34 g
Dairy	0	Fibre	5 g
Fruit	0	Salt	0.2 g
Vegetables	2		

1 medium red onion
4 spring onions
2 tsp rapeseed or other
*   neutral-tasting oil*

To serve:
120 g (4 oz) brown basmati
*   rice*

Marinate the beef for 30 minutes beforehand: if using beef sirloin, cut it into fine strips first. Slice the lemon grass stick in half lengthways, flatten the bulbous end and put it into a bowl with the juice of one of the limes. Add the beef, cover the bowl and set it aside.

Put the rice on to cook (follow the instructions on the packet). Get everything ready for the stir-fry. Cut the chilli in half, scrape out the seeds and chop it very finely.

Peel half of one side of the cucumber and then, using a potato peeler, remove several very fine strips and put them to one side. Cut the rest of the cucumber into fine batons about 4 cm (1 ½ in) long. Cut the onion in half and then slice it into fine semi-circles. Chop the spring onions finely and put some of the white parts with the thin cucumber strips.

Heat the oil in a wok or large non-stick frying pan over a high heat. Take the beef out of the bowl and shake off the lemon grass. Once the oil is almost smoking, add the beef to the wok. Stir-fry stirring constantly, for about 3 minutes, until it is cooked on all sides. Lift it out of the wok and set aside on a plate, then pour any lime juice from the marinade into the hot wok with the juice of the second lime – it will sizzle. Add the red onion, chilli, the cucumber batons and the bulk of the spring onions. Stir-fry for 2–3 minutes, until they have taken on colour and softened. Then return the beef and any juices to the wok, and stir-fry for a further minute.

Drain the rice and divide it between two plates. Put the beef stir-fry on top, then garnish with the raw cucumber strips and spring onion slices. Squeeze one of the lime skins to get a few extra drops of lime over each plate and serve immediately.

Beef meatballs with sauce

Serves 4

400 g (14 oz) lean beef mince

2 medium onions

4 garlic cloves

large sprig thyme, leaves stripped, or 1 tsp dried mixed Italian herbs

black pepper

4 tsp olive oil

200 g (7 oz) mushrooms, sliced

1 x 400 g (14 oz) tin chopped tomatoes, or a

double quantity of 'universal tomato sauce' (see page 291)

About 200 ml (7 fl oz) water

SERVINGS		NUTRITIONAL INFO	
Carbohydrate	0	Calories	256
Protein	3	Carbohydrate	10 g
Fat	½	Protein	25 g
Dairy	0	Fibre	3 g
Fruit	0	Salt	0.3 g
Vegetables	1½		

Put the mince in a bowl. Finely chop one of the onions and two of the garlic cloves and add them to the mince. Scatter the herbs over the meat and add a good grinding of black pepper, then stir everything together well with a wooden spoon. Form the mixture into 24 small balls, each about half the size of a golf ball.

Heat two teaspoons of oil in a frying pan. Carefully transfer the meatballs to the pan and brown them on all sides (this can be done in batches). Remove them from the pan and put them on a plate. Wipe the pan with a piece of kitchen paper and add the rest of the oil. Chop the remaining onion and garlic cloves, and fry them off gently until they just begun to colour. Add the mushrooms and cook for a couple of minutes – they should just begin to brown.

Pour the tomatoes or 'universal tomato sauce' into a measuring jug and add enough water or vegetable stock to make 600 ml (21 fl oz) of liquid. Transfer the onion mixture to a large saucepan, and add the tomato sauce. Carefully place the meatballs in the pan and bring the sauce to the boil, then reduce the heat to a gentle simmer, cover the pan and cook for 30 minutes. Check during this time at 10-minute intervals to ensure that the sauce isn't sticking to the bottom of the pan, and lower the heat if necessary. If the sauce seems very liquid, increase the heat a little for the final 10 minutes and take the lid off.

Tip:

▶ These meatballs are delicious with pasta or some boiled rice.

Vegetarian

Crunchy stuffed peppers with rocket and raita

Serves 2

75 g (2½ oz) long-grain
   brown rice
3 large red peppers (or one
   red, one yellow and one
   orange)
1½ tsp olive oil
1 large onion, chopped
2 garlic cloves, finely chopped

SERVINGS		NUTRITIONAL INFO	
Carbohydrate	1½	Calories	431
Protein	0	Carbohydrate	63 g
Fat	2	Protein	15 g
Dairy	½	Fibre	12 g
Fruit	0	Salt	0.2 g
Vegetables	5		

125 g (4 1/3 oz) mushrooms,
trimmed and sliced
3 tsp pine nuts
10 almonds, roughly
chopped
black pepper
100–150 ml (3½–5 fl oz)
water

For the salad:
1 bag rocket
1 tsp lemon juice

For the raita:
100 g (3½ oz) low-fat
natural yoghurt
5 cm (2 in) piece of cucumber

Cook the rice according to the packet instructions.

Preheat the oven to 190°C/375°F/Gas Mark 5. Cut the peppers in half through the stalks, and deseed them without removing the stalk (leaving the stalks on helps the peppers to hold the stuffing). Keeping them intact while removing the seeds is a bit fiddly, but using scissors makes it easier.

Put half a teaspoon of oil on a piece of kitchen paper and wipe the outside of the peppers, then put them in a baking tray, open side up. Bake for 12–15 minutes, depending on their size.

Heat the remaining teaspoon of oil in a non-stick frying pan and add the onion. Cook it for 5 minutes and then add the garlic and the mushrooms. Continue cooking for about 4 minutes, or until the mushrooms and onions are beginning to colour, then add the pine nuts, almonds and a good grinding of black pepper. Stir everything together and take the pan off the heat. Drain the cooked rice, and mix it in with the mushrooms and nuts.

Carefully lift the pepper shells off the baking tray and transfer them to an ovenproof dish (ceramic or glass). Spoon the stuffing into the shells and then pour the water around them – there should be enough to just cover the base of the dish. Put the dish in the oven and bake for 20 minutes.

Prepare the salad and yoghurt sauce while the peppers are cooking. Put the rocket leaves in a serving bowl and toss them together with the lemon juice. Spoon the yoghurt into a small bowl. Grate the cucumber into a sieve; squeeze out as much liquid as possible and then stir the cucumber into the yoghurt. When the peppers are ready, carefully lift them out of whatever water remains in the dish with a large slotted spoon and put them on serving plates. Add a generous spoonful of the yoghurt sauce and serve, accompanied by the lemony rocket. A tomato salsa is another refreshing accompaniment.

Pasta Arrabbiata (and universal tomato sauce)
Serves 2

1 red chilli, or to taste
½ tsp olive oil
1 small onion, chopped
2 garlic cloves, finely chopped
1 x 227 g (8 oz) tin chopped
   tomatoes
150 g (5 oz) dried
   wholewheat penne
basil leaves

SERVINGS		NUTRITIONAL INFO	
For Pasta Arrabbiata			
Carbohydrate	2	Calories	196
Protein	0		
Fat	0	Carbohydrate	45
Dairy	0	g Protein	10
Fruit	0	g Fibre	9 g
Vegetables	1½	Salt	0.3 g
For sauce only			
Carbohydrate	0	Calories	48
Protein	0	Carbohydrate	7 g
Fat	0	Protein	2 g
Dairy	0	Fibre	2 g
Fruit	0	Salt	0.1 g
Vegetables	1½		

Be careful when preparing chillies – cut off the top, slice the chilli in half lengthways and scrape out the seeds. Then chop the chilli finely and put it to one side.

To make the tomato sauce, heat the oil in a small pan, add the onions, garlic and chilli. Stir them together and cook very gently for about 10 minutes, or until the onion is transparent and soft. Raise the heat and add the tinned tomatoes. Simmer the sauce until it is reduced by half.

While the sauce is simmering, cook the pasta. Put a large pan of water on to boil. Cook the pasta until it is just ready – about 10 minutes.

You can either serve it as it is or as a smooth tomato sauce. If you want a smooth sauce, put a small sieve over a bowl and pour the sauce into the sieve. Push it through the sieve with a wooden spoon, and scrape the thick sauce into the bowl from the underside of the sieve. Discard the pulp, return the sauce to a clean pan and warm it through.

When the pasta is ready, drain it and put it back in the pan. Add the sauce, either as it comes or smooth, and stir thoroughly to combine. Divide it into two, scatter with a few torn basil leaves and serve.

Universal tomato sauce

For an all-purpose tomato sauce, make the sauce in the same way as described here, but leave out the chilli and include some herbs if you wish – thyme, basil and oregano are particularly good. It should generally be smooth, but that depends on how you wish to use it. It is easy to increase the quantities to make more and any extra sauce can be kept in the refrigerator for two days. It also freezes beautifully.

Tip:

▶ This pasta dish should be spicy hot, but not so hot that it's impossible to eat – and it's lightly sauced.

▶ The basic tomato sauce, without the chilli, can be used in many other recipes.

▶ Serve the pasta with cooked prawns or a sliced roast chicken breast on top.

Boston baked beans
Serves 5

2 x 400 g (14 oz) cans
  haricot or cannellini
  beans
1 tsp olive oil
1 small carrot, finely chopped
1 medium onion, finely
  chopped
1 celery stick, finely chopped
2 garlic cloves, chopped
¼ tsp cayenne pepper
1 tsp dried oregano, or a good
  handful of fresh oregano

1 x 400 g (14 oz) can
  chopped tomatoes or
  double quantity of rough
  universal tomato sauce
  (see page 291)
2 tsp honey

SERVINGS		NUTRITIONAL INFO	
Carbohydrate	0	Calories	140
Protein	1½	Carbohydrate	25 g
Fat	0	Protein	8 g
Dairy	0	Fibre	8 g
Fruit	0	Salt	0.1 g
Vegetables	1		

These beans don't have to be baked in the oven; they can be cooked on the hob as below. If it's more convenient to cook them in the oven, then preheat it to 180°C/350°F/Gas Mark 4. Just remember to check on them as they cook.

Drain and rinse the beans and put them to one side. Heat the oil in a non-stick pan and add the chopped carrot, onion and celery. Cook them gently for 10 minutes, then add the garlic and cook for another 5 minutes.

Stir in the cayenne, then add the beans and stir to combine. Add the oregano, tomatoes and honey, and cook over a medium to high heat for 20–30 minutes, stirring regularly, until much of the liquid has evaporated. When the beans are ready, check for seasoning and serve (if you are intending to freeze the beans, don't add seasoning).

Tips:

▶ Homemade baked beans are so much healthier than bought ones as they contain less salt and sugar.

▶ They freeze really well, making an ideal ready meal.

Alternative:

Soya beans give a different taste and are very useful for vegetarians as they provide a complete protein. However, they take longer to cook (you can't use the fresh ones here). Soak 200 g (7 oz) dried soya beans overnight, then rinse, cover with lots of water and boil for an hour. Lower the heat and simmer them for another hour, drain well and use as above.

Orzotto with peas and broad beans

Serves 2

1 tsp olive oil
1 small onion, chopped
1 garlic clove, finely chopped
  or crushed

80 g (2¾ oz) pearl barley
500–750 ml (17½ fl oz–1¼
  pints) hot low-salt
  vegetable stock

*100 g (3½ oz) frozen broad
beans*
100 g (3½ oz) frozen peas
black pepper

SERVINGS		NUTRITIONAL INFO	
Carbohydrate	2	Calories	259
Protein	0	Carbohydrate	48 g
Fat	0	Protein	11 g
Dairy	0	Fibre	12 g
Fruit	0	Salt	0.9 g
Vegetables	1½		

Heat the oil in a non-stick pan over a medium heat and add the chopped onion. Cook the onion and garlic gently until transparent, about 10 minutes, and then tip in the pearl barley. Stir for 2 minutes, coating it in the oil and toasting it in the hot pan, which gives it extra flavour. Then add some of the stock and let it bubble until the stock has been absorbed by the grains. Repeat this until the grains are really beginning to soften, which will take about 35–45 minutes.

When the grains are nearly done, put a pan of water on to boil. Add the broad beans, bring the pan back to the boil and simmer for a couple of minutes. Then add the peas and simmer them until both vegetables are tender. Drain well, and as soon as the barley is cooked but still has a bit of bite, add these to the pan and stir them through the orzotto. Check the seasoning, add some black papper and serve immediately.

Tips:

▶ A tangy tomato and onion salad makes a good accompaniment to this particular orzotto.

▶ You can substitute all sorts of things instead of peas and broad beans – try mushrooms or butternut squash.

▶ Pearl barley can be very variable in how long it takes to cook; some takes longer and absorbs more liquid before it finally softens and this can vary with age – the fresher the grains, the less time they take. This is why it's a good idea to cook separately anything you want to put in your orzotto, and add it to the barley at the last minute: it won't overcook.

Bean and green pepper chilli
Serves 4

2 x 400 g (14 oz) tins of
kidney beans in water
1 x 400 g (14 oz) tin of
chopped tomatoes
1 large green pepper, deseeded
and chopped
1 large onion, finely chopped
2 garlic cloves, crushed
2 tbsp tomato purée
1 tsp cayenne pepper or
chilli powder (or more,
to taste)
1 tsp ground cumin

1 tsp ground coriander
black pepper

To serve:
240 g (8 oz) basmati rice

SERVINGS		NUTRITIONAL INFO	
Carbohydrate	2	Calories	390
Protein	2	Carbohydrate	80 g
Fat	0	Protein	17 g
Dairy	0	Fibre	14 g
Fruit	0	Salt	0.2 g
Vegetables	2		

Drain and rinse the kidneys beans and put them in a large pan over a medium heat. Add the tin of tomatoes, and then the chopped pepper and onion. Add the crushed garlic to the pan, followed by the tomato purée, cayenne or chilli powder, ground cumin and coriander. Add some black pepper and stir the pan well, then cover it. Bring it to a steady simmer and cook for 30 minutes. Cook the rice according to packet instructions.

Check the chilli as it cooks and give it a stir. If there seems to be a lot of liquid, take the lid off and increase the temperature;

if it looks a little dry, add a little water. The chilli sauce should be thick rather than thin, however. Drain the rice and serve it with the chilli.

Tip:

▶ You could substitute Quorn (300 g/10½ oz) or TVP (150 g/ 5 oz) (textured vegetable protein) for one of the tins of beans.

Red pepper, courgette and mushroom lasagne
Serves 4

2 tsp olive oil
1 large onion, chopped
2 garlic cloves, finely chopped
2 red peppers, deseeded
    and chopped into 1 cm
    (¼ in) dice
1 medium courgette, sliced
    into rings
500 g (1 lb 1 oz)
    mushrooms, wiped and
    chopped
1 x 400 g (14 oz) tin
    chopped tomatoes
1 tsp dried oregano or a
    handful of fresh oregano
    leaves
8 sheets of lasagne,
    wholewheat or spinach
2 tsp grated Parmesan

SERVINGS		NUTRITIONAL INFO	
Carbohydrate	2½	Calories	374
Protein	0	Carbohydrate	50 g
Fat	1	Protein	15 g
Dairy	½	Fibre	10 g
Fruit	0	Salt	0.4 g
Vegetables	3		

For the béchamel sauce:
35 g (1¼ oz) olive oil
    margarine
35 g (1¼ oz) plain flour
350 ml (12 fl oz) skimmed
    milk
pinch of black pepper

Preheat the oven to 180°C/350°F/Gas Mark 4. Heat the olive oil in a large saucepan over a medium heat, then add the onion. Cook for 5 minutes or so, until slightly transparent. Add the garlic and stir, then add the peppers. After

5 minutes, add the courgette, mushrooms, tinned tomatoes and oregano. Cook for another 5–10 minutes, or until the vegetables are softening, then take the pan off the heat and put it to one side.

Put a large pan of water on to boil. Get out a large ovenproof dish about 6–7 cm (2½ in) deep (ideally, this should be about 25 x 25 cm/9 x 9 in, or 30 x 20 cm/11 x 7 in). Then make the sauce. Melt the margarine in a non-stick pan over a gentle heat. Once it has melted, whisk in the flour and keep whisking until it is completely mixed and starting to change colour. Then take the pan off the heat and whisk in the milk very gradually. Put the pan back on the heat and cook the sauce – still whisking – until the sauce thickens, which should only take about 3 minutes. Add a little black pepper, whisk again and then turn the heat right down or off, in the case of an electric hob. Slip the lasagne sheets into the boiling water two by two, let them soften slightly, then remove and drain on a tea towel, or use them according to the instructions on the packet.

Assemble the lasagne. Put a little of the béchamel sauce into the bottom of the ovenproof dish, then spoon about half of the vegetable mixture over it. Top with a layer of half the lasagne sheets. Then pour about half the remaining sauce on top, add another layer of vegetables, and the top with the rest of the lasagne. Pour the rest of the sauce over the pasta sheets, and sprinkle with the Parmesan. Bake in the oven for 40–45 minutes, until the top is golden and the lasagne is bubbling.

Tip:

▶ If you'd prefer not to use Parmesan, grate some Edam over the top instead.

Courgette frittata

Serves 2

2 large courgettes (about
150–175 g/5–6 oz total
weight), trimmed
2 tsp oil
1 small onion, chopped
4 eggs
black pepper

SERVINGS		NUTRITIONAL INFO	
Carbohydrate	0	Calories	233
Protein	2	Carbohydrate	4 g
Fat	½	Protein	17 g
Dairy	0	Fibre	2 g
Fruit	0	Salt	0.4 g
Vegetables	1½		

Cut the courgettes in half lengthways and then chop them into slices. Warm a teaspoon of the oil in a medium-sized frying pan, add the courgettes and onion and cook over a gentle heat until soft but not floppy. Set the pan to one side.

Beat the eggs in a bowl with some black pepper. Add the courgettes and onion to the eggs, draining off any liquid first if necessary, and mix everything together well.

Wipe the pan with some kitchen paper and put it back on the heat. Add the rest of the oil and allow it to heat, then pour in the courgette and egg mixture. Spread it out, pushing the courgette slices down with a spatula, and tilting the pan so the liquid egg runs to the edges. Cook gently, shaking the pan slightly to prevent it from sticking, for about 7 minutes or until the underside looks brown when you gently lift it up with the spatula.

Heat the grill, and put the pan under it to cook the top (let the handle stick out). Keep an eye on the frittata, as it will rise and brown quite quickly. Remove the pan from the grill, slide the frittata onto a plate and cut it into quarters. Serve immediately.

Tip:

▶ Potato wedges and steamed green beans make delicious accompaniments.

Aubergine curry with chickpeas, rice and a mango raita

Serves 4

2 medium to large aubergines (about 850 g/1 lb 14 oz total weight)

1 x 400 g (14 oz) tin of chickpeas

2 cm (½ in) square piece of fresh ginger root, peeled and finely chopped

2 garlic cloves, finely chopped

1 tbsp rapeseed or other neutral-tasting oil

1 large onion, peeled and chopped

1 red chilli, finely chopped (optional)

2 tsp garam masala

6 tbsp tomato purée

SERVINGS		NUTRITIONAL INFO	
Carbohydrate	2½	Calories	438
Protein	1	Carbohydrate	81 g
Fat	½	Protein	17 g
Dairy	½	Fibre	14 g
Fruit	0	Salt	0.5 g
Vegetables	3		

500 ml (17½ fl oz) boiling water, approximately

To serve:

240 g (8 oz) basmati rice

Mango raita:

300 g (10½ oz) low-fat natural yoghurt

2 tsp mango chutney

Cut the aubergines into slices and then cut the slices into cubes. Drain and rinse the chickpeas and set both to one side. Rinse the rice, put it in a bowl and cover with cold water. Make the raita by putting the yoghurt in a bowl and stirring in the mango chutney. Cover the bowl and put it in the refrigerator.

Chop the ginger and the garlic very finely, going over them with a knife until they are almost minced. Heat the oil in a large pan over a medium heat, and add the ginger, garlic paste and chopped onion. Cook, stirring, until the onion is soft but not beginning to colour, then add the chilli (if using) and the garam masala. Cook for a few seconds, still stirring, and then add the aubergine.

Put the tomato purée in a jug and add boiling water; stir, then pour over the aubergine until it is covered. Simmer for 10 minutes. While the aubergine is cooking, put the rice and its soaking water in a pan and cook according to the packet instructions.

When the aubergine has been cooking for 10 minutes, add the chickpeas and cover the pan. Continue cooking for another 10 minutes, keeping an eye on the level of sauce and adding a little water if necessary; give it a good stir to prevent it sticking to the bottom of the pan. If there seems to be a lot of sauce, raise the heat for the last few minutes so that some of it can cook off – this should be quite a dry dish. Serve the curry with the rice as soon as both the rice and the aubergine are ready.

Tips:

▶ The yoghurt sauce (mango raita) that accompanies this curry can also be made by adding a similar quantity of whatever Indian pickle you like, though mango works particularly well with aubergine.

▶ You can also add grated cucumber or onion to the yoghurt for a more authentic raita – squeeze excess moisture out of the cucumber first.

Sweets and Desserts

Lemon and blueberry yoghurt cake
Serves 12

200 g (7 oz) wholemeal self-raising flour
1 tsp baking powder
100 g (3½ oz) caster sugar
250 g (8⅔ oz) low-fat Greek yoghurt
50 ml (1¾ fl oz) rapeseed oil
150 ml (5 fl oz) semi-skimmed milk
juice and zest of 1 lemon

3 eggs, separated
100 g (3½ oz) blueberries

SERVINGS		NUTRITIONAL INFO	
Carbohydrate	1	Calories	174
Protein	½	Carbohydrate	23 g
Fat	½	Protein	6 g
Dairy	0	Fibre	2 g
Fruit	0	Salt	0.1 g
Vegetables	0		

Preheat the oven to 180°C /350°F/Gas Mark 4.

Lightly grease and line the base of a 20 cm (7 in) spring-form tin with baking parchment.

Sieve the flour, baking powder and caster sugar into a large bowl and make a well in the centre.

Beat together the yoghurt, oil, milk, lemon zest and juice and the egg yolks in a separate bowl. Stir in the blueberries.

In another bowl, whisk the egg whites until stiff but not dry. Pour the yoghurt mix into the dry ingredients and fold using a metal spoon, until just combined. Gently fold in the egg whites until just combined and pour the mixture into the tin. Bake in the oven for 45 minutes, until a skewer inserted into the middle comes out clean. Leave to cool in the tin for 10 minutes before turning out onto a cooling rack.

Yoghurt ice cream with raspberries
Serves 6

200 g (7 oz) very ripe raspberries, fresh or frozen
30 g (1 oz) sugar
450 g (15 oz) low-fat natural yoghurt

SERVINGS		NUTRITIONAL INFO	
Carbohydrate	½	Calories	129
Protein	0	Carbohydrate	19 g
Fat	0	Protein	7 g
Dairy	½	Fibre	3 g
Fruit	½	Salt	0.2 g
Vegetables	0		

Check over the raspberries, removing any small pieces of leaf; rinse them briefly and put them in a bowl. If using frozen berries, defrost before proceeding with the rest of the recipe. Add the sugar and stir it into the raspberries, breaking them up, then add the yoghurt. Blitz everything together using a hand-held blender (or transfer the mixture to a liquidiser).

Give the mixture a final stir to make sure it is smooth and that everything is thoroughly blended together, then pour it into a shallow freezer container or a similar dish you can safely put in the freezer. Freeze the yoghurt mixture for an hour or until crystals form around the edge. Take it out of the freezer and whisk the mixture thoroughly, then return the container to the freezer. Repeat the whisking after another hour (you can use a hand-held blender – spoon it into a bowl, blend it and return it to the freezer container), and then freeze the ice cream for at least another 2 hours, or until solid.

Take the yoghurt ice cream out of the freezer about 15 minutes before you want to serve it and leave it at room temperature to soften slightly.

Tips:

▶ You can use any berries with this recipe, as long as they are ripe and juicy.

▶ Yoghurt ice cream has a different texture to ice cream made with milk, but whisking it well helps to make it smoother.

Individual lemon and honey cheesecakes

Serves 2

3 tbsp jumbo oats

2 tsp spread, preferably sunflower

pinch ground ginger (optional)

150 g (5 oz) low-fat cream cheese, natural

1 tbsp low- or no-fat Greek yoghurt

2 tsp clear honey

zest and juice of half a large lemon

SERVINGS		NUTRITIONAL INFO	
Carbohydrate	2	Calories	213
Protein	0	Carbohydrate	23 g
Fat	1	Protein	12 g
Dairy	2½	Fibre	2 g
Fruit	0	Salt	0.9 g
Vegetables	0		

Put the oats into a dry pan over a medium heat. Stir with a wooden spoon until they suddenly start to smell toasty and change colour. Take the pan off the heat, empty the oats into a small bowl, then add the spread and the ground ginger (if using). Mix these together immediately, working the spread in with a wooden spoon; the warmth of the oats will melt it. When thoroughly combined, divide the mixture between two ramekins (or 2 wine or spirit glasses) and press it into the base. Put the ramekins in the refrigerator for at least an hour.

Take the cream cheese out of the refrigerator 10 minutes before you make the filling so that it is soft enough to work with. Put the cheese, yoghurt and honey in a bowl and beat them together. Add the lemon juice and beat that in, too. Carefully divide the mixture between the two ramekins. Level the tops, and put them back in the refrigerator for another 3 hours (or more). Just before serving, scatter the top of each cheesecake with the lemon zest.

Crunchy blackberry and apple crumble
Serves 4

320 g (11 oz) dessert apples
squeeze of lemon juice
320 g (11 oz) ripe
  blackberries

For the crumble topping:
125 g (4 1/3 oz) porridge oats
25 g (¾ oz) ground almonds
25 g (¾ oz) wholemeal flour
25 g (¾ oz) light brown
  sugar

50 g (1¾ oz) olive oil spread
  or similar
½ tsp cinnamon

SERVINGS		NUTRITIONAL INFO	
Carbohydrate	1½	Calories	326
Protein	0	Carbohydrate	46 g
Fat	2	Protein	7 g
Dairy	0	Fibre	10 g
Fruit	2	Salt	0.3 g
Vegetables	0		

Preheat the oven to 180°C/350°F/Gas Mark 4. Peel, core and chop the apples and put them in a bowl. Squeeze over some lemon juice, then add the blackberries and mix these together well. Tip the fruit into a medium-sized ovenproof dish (about 18–20 cm/7–8 in diameter).

Put the oats, ground almonds, flour and brown sugar in a bowl and mix them together. Then add the spread and rub it in until the mixture resembles fine breadcrumbs. Add the cinnamon and mix it in too. Spoon the crumble over the fruit and press it down. Put the dish in the oven and bake it for about 30–40 minutes, or until the top is golden brown. Serve with low or no-fat Greek yoghurt.

Crêpes

Serves 4 (makes 4 crêpes, using a medium frying pan)

85 g (3 oz) plain flour
1 tbsp wholemeal flour
1 medium egg
250 ml (8½ fl oz) semi-
  skimmed milk
1 tsp sunflower spread per
  crêpe

To serve:
juice of 1 lemon
4 tsp clear honey

SERVINGS		NUTRITIONAL INFO	
Crêpes			
Carbohydrate	1	Calories	166
Protein	0	Carbohydrate	23 g
Fat	1	Protein	7 g
Dairy	0	Fibre	1 g
Fruit	0	Salt	0.2 g
Vegetables	0		
With Honey			
Carbohydrate	1½	Calories	189
Protein	0	Carbohydrate	29 g
Fat	1	Protein	7 g
Dairy	0	Fibre	1 g
Fruit	0	Salt	0.2 g
Vegetables	0		

Put the flours into a bowl and break in the egg. Using a whisk, stir these together, breaking up the yolk, then gradually add the milk, whisking until you have a mixture the consistency of single cream without lumps.

Put a non-stick frying pan over a high heat. When the pan is hot, add a little spread and let it melt; tip the pan to spread it over the surface. Now add the batter – about 3–4 tablespoons per crêpe, though this will depend on the size of pan: crêpes should be thinner than standard pancakes. Again tip the pan in all directions, letting the batter run to the sides. Put it back on the heat and, after a couple of minutes cooking, gently lift one side of the crepe: it should be lightly browned. Flip it over (a fish slice or palette knife is useful) and cook the underside – this will take less time; allow a minute.

You can either make one crêpe and store the rest of the batter in the refrigerator, or you can make the whole batch. If making all four in one go, once the first crêpe is cooked, slide it onto a warm plate, cover lightly with foil and keep warm in a coolish oven while you continue. Once ready to eat, slide the crêpe onto a serving plate, drizzle with lemon juice and a teaspoon of clear honey, and roll it over. Serve immediately.

Tip:
▶ Instead of honey, serve with chopped banana or mixed berries and a spoon of low-fat Greek yoghurt.

Apricot and apple fruit salad
Serves 2

4 dried apricots, chopped
50 ml (1¾ fl oz) apple juice, chilled
4 fresh apricots
2 small dessert apples

SERVINGS		NUTRITIONAL INFO	
Carbohydrate	0	Calories	94
Protein	0	Carbohydrate	23 g
Fat	0	Protein	2 g
Dairy	0	Fibre	5 g
Fruit	2	Salt	<0.1 g
Vegetables	0		

Put the dried apricots in a bowl. Add the apple juice, cover the bowl and leave it in the refrigerator for at least an hour. Cut up the fresh apricots: halve and remove the stones first, then chop into smaller pieces and add them to the bowl. Cut the apples into fine slices and stir these in. Divide the fruit between two serving bowls and spoon over any apple juice that remains in the larger bowl. Serve immediately.

Tip:
▶ Fresh apricots are delicious, but very seasonal. If you can't find them, choose ripe plums instead.

Baked nectarines stuffed with nuts
Serves 2

2 ripe nectarines
2 level tbsp ground almonds
1 tsp sugar
15 almonds, chopped
1 tsp shelled unsalted

pistachios, chopped (optional, if not using, add 5 more almonds)
100 ml (3½ fl oz) orange juice

Preheat the oven to 200°C/ 400°F/Gas Mark 6. You will need a small ovenproof dish just big enough to hold four halves of nectarine so that they don't topple over.

SERVINGS		NUTRITIONAL INFO	
Carbohydrate	0	Calories	219
Protein	0	Carbohydrate	18 g
Fat	3	Protein	7 g
Dairy	0	Fibre	4 g
Fruit	1½	Salt	<0.1 g
Vegetables	0		

Halve the nectarines, cutting through to the stone. Twist one half of each fruit to release it from the stone, and then cut the stone out of the other half. Place the halves in the ovenproof dish, cut side uppermost.

Put the ground almonds into a bowl and add the sugar and chopped nuts, then moisten the mixture with a little orange juice until it holds together. Mix well, and then spoon it into the cavities left by the nectarine stones. Pour the rest of the orange juice into the dish around the fruit.

Cover the dish lightly with foil and put it into the oven. Bake for 15 minutes, then remove the foil. Cook for another 5 minutes, or until soft. Gently lift each fruit out of the oven- proof dish with a slotted spoon, and put it in a serving bowl. Spoon a little of the juice around each, and serve immediately.

Chocolate and orange mousse

NB: This recipe contains raw eggs and is therefore not suitable to be shared with anyone who is pregnant or in poor health.
Serves 4

*125 g (4 1/3 oz) dark
    chocolate, at least 70%
    cocoa solids*

*1 small orange
3 medium eggs*

Sit a glass heatproof bowl over a pan so that it sits above the pan without touching the bottom; it should be clear by at least 3 cm (1 in). You will also need four small glasses or ramekins.

SERVINGS		NUTRITIONAL INFO	
Carbohydrate	2	Calories	245
Protein	1	Carbohydrate	24 g
Fat	2	Protein	8 g
Dairy	0	Fibre	3 g
Fruit	0	Salt	0.2 g
Vegetables	0		

Break the chocolate into small pieces and put it in the bowl. Zest and juice the orange, then set the zest to one side. Add most of the orange juice to the bowl with the chocolate. Put about 1.5 cm (½ in) of water into the pan and bring it to a steady simmer over a medium heat. Place the bowl over, but not touching, the water (double-check that it isn't touching the surface), and allow the chocolate to melt, stirring it with a wooden spoon.

Separate the eggs, and put the whites in another bowl. Whisk the whites until they form soft peaks using an electric whisk if possible, by which time the chocolate should have melted. Take the bowl off the pan and add the rest of the orange juice.

Tip in the egg yolks and beat them in, working energetically. When the egg yolks are all combined and the chocolate has a lovely glossy appearance, add some of the whisked egg white. Using a metal spoon, gently fold it in until the mixture is a uniform colour, and then repeat until all the white has been added. Now carefully spoon the chocolate mousse into the glasses or ramekins, tap them on the worktop to level them off, and then put them in the refrigerator to chill for at least 5 hours or overnight.

Just before serving, scatter some of the reserved orange zest over each one.

Tips:

▶ A few fresh raspberries on the side makes a lovely addition.

▶ This healthier version of a classic dish is still deliciously rich (you may find that it will stretch to 6 servings).

▶ It is adaptable: you could use strong black coffee instead of the orange juice, for instance. You'll need about 4 tablespoons in total.

Prune delight
Serves 4

200 g (7 oz) pitted prunes
1 tbsp clear honey
250 g (8 2/3 oz) low- or
no-fat Greek yoghurt

SERVINGS		NUTRITIONAL INFO	
Carbohydrate	1	Calories	147
Protein	0	Carbohydrate	29 g
Fat	0	Protein	5 g
Dairy	½	Fibre	4 g
Fruit	1½	Salt	0.1 g
Vegetables	0		

Put the prunes into a bowl and pour over a mugful of water; stir, cover and set it aside. Soak them overnight or for several hours.

Empty the prunes and their soaking liquid into a pan over a high heat and bring them to the boil. Then lower the heat and simmer for about 15 minutes, by which time they should be starting to fall apart. Purée them with a hand-held blender or food processor and transfer to a clean bowl; alternatively, push the cooked prunes through a sieve into the bowl with a wooden spoon. Set the prune purée aside and allow it to cool.

Mix the honey and the yoghurt together well, then spoon this mixture into the cooled prunes. Stir together thoroughly and then transfer the mixture into a serving bowl, or into individual ramekins or glasses. Chill for at least an hour before serving.

Tip:

▶ For a fragrant flavour variation, use a scented tea such as Earl Grey as the soaking liquid.

Apple fool with heather honey
Serves 4

3 large cooking apples
pinch of cinnamon, to taste
*   (optional)*
juice of 1 orange
2 tsp heather honey, or
*   similarly strongly*
*   flavoured honey*
300 g (10½ oz) low- or
*   no-fat Greek yoghurt*

SERVINGS		NUTRITIONAL INFO	
Carbohydrate	½	Calories	122
Protein	0	Carbohydrate	22 g
Fat	0	Protein	5 g
Dairy	½	Fibre	1 g
Fruit	2	Salt	0.2 g
Vegetables	0		

Peel, core and chop the cooking apples and put them straight into a pan with a little water – no more than 50 ml (1¾ fl oz). Add the cinnamon, if using, and the orange juice. Simmer the apples gently until they are really soft, stirring to ensure they don't stick to the bottom of the pan. Remove the pan from the heat and allow the apples to cool down, then blend them until smooth. Spoon the apple purée into a large bowl, cover it with cling film and chill in the fridge for at least an hour.

Once the purée is thoroughly chilled, add the honey and the yoghurt. Gently fold these into the apple purée, then spoon it into serving dishes. These can either be served immediately or can be put back in the fridge to chill once more, and be used later.

Hosaf – Turkish dried fruit salad
Serves 2

6 stoned prunes
6 dried apricots
2 tsp sultanas
1 tsp pine nuts
1 tsp unsalted pistachios,
    chopped (optional)
1 tbsp flaked almonds

SERVINGS		NUTRITIONAL INFO	
Protein	0	Calories	249
Fat	1½	Carbohydrate	30 g
Dairy	0	Protein	7 g
Fruit	2	Fibre	7 g
Vegetables	0	Salt	<0.1 g

Put the prunes, apricots, sultanas and pine nuts in a small pan, with enough water to just cover everything. Stir well and put the pan on a medium heat. Simmer the fruit gently for 20–25 minutes, then empty into a bowl and allow it to cool down for a couple of hours (or even overnight). Put the Hosaf into 2 serving dishes and scatter the almonds and pistachios over it just before serving.

Tip:
▶ Traditionally the pine nuts should be soft. If you prefer them crunchier add them at the end with the almonds and pistachios.

final word

Some of the Dieters who started The 2-Day Diet had never tried to lose weight before, but many of them had tried over and over again – sometimes losing weight, but mainly putting it back on. Their success with this new diet – which amazed many of them and delighted us – proved to us that there is another way to lose weight and keep it off for good. If you are one of those people, or you simply want an alternative to the grind of a seven-day diet, The 2-Day Diet can work for you. The formula is a simple one: two days of restricted high-protein, low-carb eating, five days of an unrestricted healthy Mediterranean diet and regular exercise. We know it's not a quick fix and it may take a while for you to adjust your eating habits, but we believe that this is a truly innovative – and healthy – approach to weight loss. We will continue with our research to understand more about the particular health benefits of this diet and this type of weight loss, but in the meantime we hope that The 2-Day Diet will be the approach that works for you. Follow the Diet, get going on an exercise programme and when you've lost your weight, stay with The 1-Day Maintenance Diet and you will achieve the healthy weight and the healthy body you have been hoping for.

appendices

Appendix A:
How much body fat do I have?

Female Body Fat Percentage Ready Reckoner

BMI	Age											
	18	20	25	30	35	40	45	50	55	60	65	70
18	20	20	21	22	23	24	26	27	28	29	30	31
19	22	22	23	24	25	26	27	28	29	30	31	32
20	24	24	25	26	27	28	29	30	31	32	33	33
21	26	26	27	28	29	29	30	31	32	33	34	35
22	27	28	29	29	30	31	32	33	34	34	35	36
23	29	30	30	31	32	33	33	34	35	36	36	37
24	31	31	32	33	33	34	35	36	36	37	38	38
25	33	33	34	34	35	36	36	37	38	38	39	40
26	34	34	35	36	36	37	38	38	39	39	40	41
27	36	36	37	37	38	38	39	39	40	41	41	42
28	37	37	38	39	39	40	40	41	41	42	42	43
29	39	39	39	40	40	41	41	42	42	43	43	44
30	40	40	41	41	42	42	43	43	43	44	44	45
31	41	42	42	42	43	43	44	44	45	45	45	46
32	43	43	43	44	44	44	45	45	46	46	46	47
33	44	44	44	45	45	45	46	46	47	47	47	48
34	45	45	46	46	46	46	47	47	47	48	48	48
35	46	46	47	47	47	47	48	48	48	49	49	49
36	47	47	48	48	48	48	49	49	49	50	50	50
37	48	48	49	49	49	49	50	50	50	50	51	51
38	49	49	50	50	50	50	50	51	51	51	51	52
39	50	50	50	51	51	51	51	51	52	52	52	52
40	51	51	51	51	52	52	52	52	52	53	53	53

To find your body fat percentage you go down to your BMI score and then across to your closest age. You can calculate your BMI on page 31.

For example a female who has a BMI of 22 and is 42 years old has a body fat percentage of 31%.

Male Body Fat Percentage Ready Reckoner

BMI	Age											
	18	20	25	30	35	40	45	50	55	60	65	70
18	11	11	12	13	14	15	16	17	19	20	21	22
19	13	13	14	15	16	17	18	19	20	21	22	23
20	15	15	16	17	18	19	20	21	22	23	24	25
21	17	17	18	19	20	21	22	23	24	24	25	26
22	19	19	20	21	22	23	24	24	25	26	27	28
23	21	21	22	23	24	25	25	26	27	28	28	29
24	23	23	24	25	26	26	27	28	28	29	30	31
25	25	25	26	27	27	28	29	29	30	31	31	32
26	27	27	28	28	29	30	30	31	31	32	33	33
27	29	29	29	30	31	31	32	32	33	34	34	35
28	30	31	31	32	32	33	33	34	34	35	36	36
29	32	32	33	33	34	34	35	35	36	36	37	37
30	34	34	35	35	35	36	36	37	37	38	38	39
31	35	36	36	37	37	37	38	38	39	39	39	40
32	37	37	38	38	38	39	39	40	40	40	41	41
33	39	39	39	39	40	40	41	41	41	42	42	42
34	40	40	41	41	41	42	42	42	43	43	43	44
35	42	42	42	42	43	43	43	44	44	44	44	45
36	43	43	43	44	44	44	45	45	45	45	46	46
37	44	44	45	45	45	45	46	46	46	47	47	47
38	46	46	46	46	47	47	47	47	47	48	48	48
39	47	47	47	48	48	48	48	48	49	49	49	49
40	48	48	49	49	49	49	49	49	50	50	50	50

To find your body fat percentage you go down to your BMI score and then across to your closest age. You can calculate your BMI on page 31.

For example a male who has a BMI of 22 and is 42 years old has a body fat percentage of 23%.

Ready reckoner based on CUN-BAE equation[1].

Women should have between 20% and 34% of their body weight as fat, men 8–25%[2].

Appendix B: How much can I eat on each of my two restricted days?

The food lists below show how much you can eat on each restricted day. If you feel full you do not have to eat the maximum fat servings. Try to eat the minimum protein and all of your vegetable, dairy and fruit allowance. For detailed information including variations for vegetarians see Chapter 3.

Carbohydrate foods	Carbohydrate foods
Carbohydrates are not allowed on your two restricted diet days of The 2-Day Diet	0 servings

Protein	1 serving (uncooked) equal to:
Women: minimum 4–maximum 12 servings Men: minimum 4–maximum 14 servings	
Fresh or smoked white fish, e.g. haddock or cod	60 g (2 oz) (two fish-finger sized pieces)
Seafood, e.g. prawns, mussels, crab	45 g (1½ oz)
Tinned tuna in brine or spring water	45 g (1½ oz)
Oily fish (fresh or tinned) in tomato sauce or oil (drained), for example, mackerel, sardines, salmon, trout, tuna, smoked salmon* or trout* or kippers*	30 g (1 oz)
Chicken, turkey, duck, pheasant (cooked without skin)	30 g (1 oz) (a slice the size of a playing card)
Lean beef, pork, lamb, rabbit, venison, offal	30 g (1 oz) per serving to a maximum of 500 g (1 lb 1 oz) per week for women and 600 g (1 lb 4 oz) per week for men (including the two restricted days and five unrestricted days of The 2-Day Diet)
Lean bacon*	1 grilled rasher
Lean ham*	2 medium or 4 wafer-thin slices

* see page 55

Protein	1 serving (uncooked) equal to:
Eggs	1 medium/large egg
Tofu	50 g (1¾ oz)

Include only one of the below on each restricted day. They count towards your daily protein allowance.

Protein	Maximum	Servings
Textured vegetable protein (TVP)	maximum 30 g (1 oz) per day	3
Soya and edamame beans	maximum 60 g (2 oz) per day	2
Low-fat hummus	maximum 1 heaped tablespoon (30 g/1 oz) per day	1
Quorn	maximum 115 g (4 oz) per day	4
Vegetarian sausage	1 sausage	2

Fat	1 serving equal to:
Women: maximum 5 servings Men: maximum 6 servings	
Margarine or low-fat spread (avoid the 'buttery' types)	1 teaspoon (8 g)
Olive oil or other oil (not palm, coconut or ghee)	1 dessertspoon (7 g)
Oil-based dressing	1 dessertspoon (7 g)
Unsalted or salted* or dry roasted nuts (not honey roast), seeds (e.g. sesame or linseed)	1 dessertspoon per serving or 3 walnut halves, 3 Brazil nuts, 4 almonds, 8 peanuts, 10 cashews or 10 pistachios (not chestnuts)
Pesto	1 teaspoon (8 g)
Mayonnaise	1 teaspoon (5 g)
Low-fat mayonnaise	1 tablespoon (15 g)
Olives*	10
Peanut or other nut butter (without palm oil)	1 teaspoon (8 g)

* see page 55

The 2-Day Diet

You can only have one of the following fatty foods on each restricted day as they contain some carbohydrate. They count towards your fat serving allowance.

Fat	Maximum	Servings
Avocado	½ pear	2
Guacamole	2 tablespoons	2
Low-fat Guacamole	2 tablespoons	1

Dairy (3 servings per day for all)	1 serving equal to:
Milk (semi-skimmed or skimmed)	200 ml (⅓ pint/7 fl oz)
Soya milk (sweetened or unsweetened with added calcium)	200 ml (⅓ pint/7 fl oz)
Yoghurt: diet fruit, plain soya; Greek, plain or fromage frais (all low fat)	1 small pot 120–150 g (4–5 oz) or 3 heaped tablespoons
Whole milk plain yoghurt	80–90 g or 2 heaped tablespoons
Cottage cheese	75 g (2½ oz) or 2 tablespoons
Quark	⅓ pot or 3 tablespoons (90 g/3 oz)
Cream cheese (light or extra-light)	1 tablespoon (30 g/1 oz)
Lower-fat cheeses: reduced-fat Cheddar, Edam, Bavarian smoked, feta*, Camembert, ricotta, mozzarella, reduced-fat halloumi	Matchbox size – 30 g (1 oz) per serving to a maximum of 120 g (4 oz) for women per week and 150 g (5 oz) for men on restricted and un-restricted days

Vegetables (5 servings per day for all)	1 serving equal to:
Artichoke	2 globe hearts
Asparagus, tinned	7 spears
Asparagus, fresh	5 spears
Aubergine	⅓ medium

* see page 55

Vegetables continued	1 serving equal to:
Beans, French	4 heaped tablespoons
Beans, runner	4 heaped tablespoons
Beansprouts, fresh	2 handfuls
Broccoli	2 spears
Brussels sprouts	8
Cabbage	⅙ small cabbage or 3 heaped tablespoons shredded leaves
Cauliflower	8 florets
Celeriac	3 heaped tablespoons
Celery	3 sticks
Chinese leaves	⅕ 'head'
Courgette	½ large courgette
Cucumber	5 cm (2 in) piece
Curly kale, cooked	4 heaped tablespoons
Fennel	½ cup sliced
Karela or gourd	½
Leeks	1 medium
Lettuce (mixed leaves or rocket)	1 cereal bowlful
Mangetout	1 handful
Mushrooms, fresh	14 button or 3 handfuls of slices
Mushrooms, dried	2 tablespoons or handful porcini
Okra	16 medium
Pak choi (Chinese cabbage)	2 handfuls
Pepper (green only)	½
Pumpkin	3 heaped tablespoons

The 2-Day Diet

Vegetables continued	1 serving equal to:
Radish	10
Spinach, cooked	2 heaped tablespoons
Spinach, fresh	1 cereal bowlful
Spring greens, cooked	4 heaped tablespoons
Spring onion	8
Sweetcorn, baby (whole not kernels)	6
Tomato, tinned	2 plum tomatoes or ½ tin chopped
Tomato, fresh	1 medium or 7 cherry
Tomato purée	1 heaped tablespoon
Tomato, sundried	4 pieces
Watercress	1 cereal bowlful

Fruit (1 serving per day for all)	1 serving equal to:
Apricots	3 fresh or dried
Blackberries	1 handful
Blackcurrants	4 heaped tablespoons
Redcurrants	4 heaped tablespoons
Grapefruit, guava	½ whole fruit
Melon	5 cm (2 in) slice
Pineapple	1 large slice
Peach	1 fruit
Papaya	1 slice
Passion fruit	5 fruits
Raspberries	2 handfuls
Strawberries	7

Fruit (1 serving per day for all)	1 serving equal to:
Stewed rhubarb, gooseberries or cranberries,with sweetener	3 heaped tablespoons

Flavourings	1 serving equal to:
Lemon juice; fresh or dried herbs; spices; black pepper; mustard, horseradish, vinegars, garlic, fresh or pre-chopped; chilli, fresh or dried; soy sauce; miso paste; fish sauce; Worcester sauce	Unlimited

Drinks	At least 8 drinks or 2 litres (4 pints) a day
Water (still or sparkling)	Unlimited
Tea and coffee, caffeinated or decaffeinated	Unlimited
Fruit, herbal or green teas	Unlimited
Sugar-free or diet squash or fizzy drinks (3 litres/6 pints) per week	Up to a maximum of 9 cans

Appendix C: How much can I eat on each unrestricted day of The 2-Day Diet?

We encourage you to follow a healthy Mediterranean diet on your unrestricted days. This allows you a wider range of foods than your two restricted days and includes carbohydrates, protein, low-fat dairy foods and a wide range of fruits and vegetables. The tables below are a guide to what makes up a single serving of a given food. You are allowed different numbers of servings from each food group, depending on your gender, weight and age. The tables in Appendix D will advise the right quantity of these servings for you. For detailed information on the Mediterranean diet please refer to Chapter 4.

Carbohydrate foods (amounts vary – check the ready reckoner)	1 serving equal to:
Wholewheat or oat breakfast cereal	3 level tablespoons (24 g/¾ oz), or 1 wholewheat or oat bisk
Porridge oats or sugar-free muesli	1 heaped tablespoon (20 g/⅔ oz)
Wholegrain, wholemeal, rye, granary bread	Medium slice, ½ roll
Pitta bread, chapatti, tortilla wrap (wholemeal or multigrain versions)	½ large
Rye crispbread	2
Wholewheat cracker	2
Oat cake (choose a variety without palm oil)	1
Dried wholegrain pasta or rice	1 tablespoon uncooked (30 g/1 oz) or 2 tablespoons cooked (60 g/2 oz)
Couscous, bulgur wheat, pearl barley, quinoa	1 tablespoon uncooked (30 g/1 oz) or 2 tablespoons cooked (60 g/2 oz)
Lasagne (preferably wholemeal)	1 sheet

appendices

Carbohydrate foods continued	1 serving equal to:
Noodles (preferable brown)	Half a dried block or nest (50 g/1¾ oz)
Baked or boiled potato (in skin)	1 small (120 g/4 oz) raw weight
Cassava, yam, sweet potato	1 small (90 g/3 oz) raw weight
Wholemeal pizza base	⅙ of thin medium pizza base
Sweet corn	½ corn on the cob or 2 tablespoons kernels
Wholemeal flour	Level tablespoon
Unsweetened popcorn	20 g (⅔ oz)

Protein foods (amounts vary – check the ready reckoner)	1 serving (uncooked) equal to:
Fresh or smoked* white fish (for example, haddock or cod)	60 g (2 oz) (two fish finger sized pieces)
Tinned tuna in brine or spring water	45 g (1½ oz)
Oily fish (fresh or tinned) in tomato sauce or oil (drained), for example, mackerel, sardines, salmon, trout, tuna, smoked salmon* or trout* or kippers*	30 g (1 oz)
Seafood, e.g. prawns, mussels, crab	45 g (1½ oz)
Chicken, turkey or duck (cooked without the skin)	30 g (1 oz) (a slice the size of a playing card)
Lean beef, pork, lamb, rabbit, venison or offal (fat removed)	30 g (1 oz) per serving to a maximum of 500 g (1 lb 1 oz) per week for women and 600 g (1 lb 4 oz) per week for men
Lean bacon*	1 rasher
Ham*	2 medium slices or 4 wafer-thin slices
Eggs	1 medium/large
Baked beans	2 level tablespoons (60 g/2 oz)

* Try to have these salty foods only once during your five unrestricted days

The 2-Day Diet

Protein foods continued	1 serving equal to:
Lentils, chickpeas and beans	1 tablespoon (20 g/ 2/3 oz) raw or 1½ tablespoons cooked or tinned (65 g/2 oz)
Quorn, e.g. pieces, mince, fillets	30 g (1 oz)
Vegetarian sausage	½
Tofu	⅛ of packet (50 g/1¾ oz)
Textured vegetable protein (TVP)	1 heaped tablespoon (10 g/ ⅓ oz) uncooked
Frozen vegetarian mince	30 g (1 oz)
Low-fat hummus	1 heaped tablespoon (30 g/1 oz)

Fat (amounts vary – check the ready reckoner)	1 serving equal to:
Margarine or low-fat spread, avoid the buttery types)	1 teaspoon (8 g)
Olive oil or other oil	1 dessertspoon (7 g)
Oil based dressing	1 dessertspoon (7 g)
Unsalted nuts/seeds (e.g. sesame, linseed)	1 dessertspoon or 3 walnut halves, 3 Brazil nuts, 4 almonds, 8 peanuts, 10 cashews or pistachios
Avocado	¼ average pear
Pesto	1 level teaspoon (8 g)
Olives*	10
Mayonnaise	1 teaspoon (5 g)
Guacamole or low-fat mayonnaise	1 tablespoon (15 g)
Low-fat guacamole	2 tablespoons (30 g)
Peanut butter (choose a variety without palm oil)	1 heaped teaspoon (11 g)

* Try to have these salty foods only once during your five unrestricted days

Milk and dairy foods (3 servings per day for all)	1 serving equal to:
Milk (semi-skimmed or skimmed)	200 ml (⅓ pint/7 fl oz)
Alternative 'milks', e.g. soya, oat (sweetened or unsweetened)	200 ml (⅓ pint/7 fl oz)
Reduced-fat evaporated milk	1 level tablespoon (15 g)
Yoghurt: diet fruit, plain soya; Greek, plain or fromage frais (all low fat)	1 small pot (120–150 g/4–5 oz) or 3 heaped tablespoons
Yoghurt: low-fat fruit, whole milk fruit and plain, flavoured soya yoghurt	80–90 g (2½–3 oz) or 2 heaped tablespoons
Cottage cheese	¼ pot (75 g/2½ oz) or 2 tablespoons
Cream cheese (light or extra-light)	1 level tablespoon (30 g/1 oz)
Quark	⅓ pot or 3 level tablespoons (90 g/3 oz)
Lower-fat cheeses: Reduced fat Cheddar, Edam, Bavarian smoked, feta*, Camembert, ricotta, mozzarella, reduced-fat halloumi	Matchbox-sized 30 g (1 oz). No more than 120 g (4 oz) per week for women and 150 g (5 oz) for men.

Vegetables (at least 5 servings per day for all)	1 serving equal to 80 g (2½ oz)
Any boiled or steamed vegetables (Except potato, yam, sweet corn, which are carbohydrates or pulses, which are counted as protein.)	2–3 heaped tablespoons
Salad	1 bowl
Homemade vegetable soup	½ bowl
Vegetable juice†	200 ml (⅓ pint/7 fl oz)
Tomato purée	1 level tablespoon

† Limit to 1 glass of fruit and vegetable juice per day

* see page 55

The 2-Day Diet

Fruit (all varieties allowed – 1 serving per day for all)	1 serving equal to:
Banana	1 small
Berries: e.g. blueberries, blackberries, redcurrants, raspberries, strawberries	1 cup (80 g/2½ oz)
Dried fruit	3 dried apricots, small figs, small dates/handful raisins
Fruit juice	Small glass (125 ml/4 fl oz)[†]
Grapes, cherries	15
Grapefruit, guava	½ whole fruit
Mango, melon, pineapple, papaya	1 slice (80 g/2½ oz)
Apple, kiwi, nectarine, orange, peach, pear, pomegranate, Sharon fruit	1 fruit
Small fruits: e.g. apricots, clementines, dates (fresh), figs (fresh), passion fruit, plums	2 fruits
Any stewed fruit (unsweetened or with sweetener). e.g. apple, cranberry, rhubarb	3 level tablespoons
Any tinned fruit (in natural juice)	3 level tablespoons
Prepacked fruit salads	80 g/2½ oz
Kumquats, lychees, physalis	5 fruits

[†] Limit to 1 glass of fruit and vegetable juice per day

Drinks	At least 8 drinks or 2 litres (4 pints) a day
Water (still or sparkling)	Unlimited
Tea and coffee, caffeinated or decaffeinated	Unlimited
Fruit, herbal or green teas	Unlimited
Sugar-free or diet squash or fizzy drinks	Up to a maximum of 9 cans (3 litres/6 pints) per week

Drinks	At least 8 drinks or 2 litres (4 pints) a day
Alcohol	Up to a maximum of 10 units (100 g) a week (see page 87)

Treats (up to 3 servings a week on unrestricted days)	Treat serving:
Low-fat crisps	1 small packet (25–30 g/¾–1 oz)
Plain or chocolate biscuits (e.g. digestive)	2
Chocolate (ideally dark 70% cocoa or higher content)	5 small squares or 30 g (1 oz)
Ice cream	2 scoops standard or 1 scoop luxury
Malt loaf	1 slice
Hot cross bun	1 bun
Fruity teacake	1 teacake
Fairy cakes	2 small cakes with thin or no icing
Flapjack	2 'mini bites' (3 cm/1 in square)
Jaffa cakes or small chocolate chip cookies	3
Individual chocolate or truffle	3

Appendix D: Quick reference to how much I can eat

Use these tables to look up how many calories or servings of foods you can have a day according to your gender, age and weight. They include both information for weight loss and information for weight maintenance.

- Energy requirements have been determined using the Henry equations[3] based on your gender, age and weight. You will lose weight quicker if you also follow the exercise recommendations in the book.
- It is important to get adequate protein, dairy, fruit and vegetables on the two restricted and five unrestricted days of The 2-Day Diet. This is why there are minimum amounts for protein, and recommended amounts for dairy, fruit and vegetables each day. These meal plans have been designed so you will achieve the recommended amount of 1.2 g of protein per kilogram of body weight each day[4].
- You do not need to eat the maximum amounts in the table. However, it is important to get the balance of foods right. For example if you only have two-thirds of your maximum protein servings you should also roughly aim for two-thirds of your maximum fat and high-fibre carbohydrate servings.
- Try to get 24 g of fibre on each unrestricted day (see page 336).

Ready reckoner | Weight loss | Males

Up to 12½ stone (79 kg)

	2 restricted days	5 unrestricted days														
		Less than 8½ stone (54 kg)			8½–9½ stone (54–60 kg)			9½–10½ stone (60–67 kg)			10½–11½ stone (67–73 kg)			11½–12½ stone (73–79 kg)		
		Age 18–29	Age 30–60	Age 60+	Age 18–29	Age 30–60	Age 60+	Age 18–29	Age 30–60	Age 60+	Age 18–29	Age 30–60	Age 60+	Age 18–29	Age 30–60	Age 60+
Maximum kcal per day	1,100	1,600	1,600	1,400	1,700	1,600	1,400	1,900	1,800	1,600	2,000	1,900	1,700	2,100	2,000	1,800
Carbohydrate servings	0	Max 7	Max 7	Max 6	Max 7	Max 7	Max 6	Max 8	Max 8	Max 7	Max 9	Max 9	Max 7	Max 11	Max 9	Max 8
Protein servings	Min 4	Min 3	Min 3	Min 3	Min 4	Min 4	Min 4	Min 5	Min 5	Min 5	Min 6	Min 6	Min 6	Min 7	Min 7	Min 7
	Max 14	Max 9	Max 9	Max 8	Max 10	Max 9	Max 8	Max 12	Max 11	Max 9	Max 14	Max 12	Max 10	Max 14	Max 14	Max 11
Fat servings	Max 6	Max 4	Max 4	Max 3	Max 5	Max 4	Max 3	Max 5	Max 5	Max 4	Max 5	Max 5	Max 5	Max 5	Max 5	Max 5
Dairy servings	3 (recommended)	3 (recommended for all weight groups)														
Vegetable servings	5 (recommended)	5 (recommended for all weight groups)														
Fruit servings	1 (recommended)	2 (recommended for all weight groups)														

Ready reckoner | Weight loss | Males
Over 12½ stone (79 kg)

	2 restricted days	5 unrestricted days											
		12½–13½ stone (79–86 kg)			13½–14½ stone (86–92 kg)			14½–15½ stone (92–98 kg)			Above 15½ stone (98 kg)		
		Age 18–29	Age 30–60	Age 60+	Age 18–29	Age 30–60	Age 60+	Age 18–29	Age 30–60	Age 60+	Age 18–29	Age 30–60	Age 60+
Maximum kcal per day	1,100	2,300	2,200	2,000	2,500	2,300	2,100	2,500	2,400	2,200	2,500	2,500	2,300
Carbohydrate servings	0	Max 12	Max 11	Max 9	Max 13	Max 12	Max 11	Max 13	Max 12	Max 11	Max 13	Max 13	Max 12
Protein servings	Min 4	Min 8	Min 8	Min 8	Min 9	Min 9	Min 9	Min 10	Min 10	Min 10	Min 11	Min 11	Min 11
	Max 14	Max 16	Max 15	Max 14	Max 17	Max 16	Max 14	Max 17	Max 17	Max 15	Max 17	Max 17	Max 16
Fat servings	Max 6	Max 6	Max 5	Max 5	Max 7	Max 6	Max 5	Max 7	Max 6	Max 5	Max 7	Max 7	Max 6
Dairy servings	3 (recommended)	3 (recommended for all weight groups)											
Vegetable servings	5 (recommended)	5 (recommended for all weight groups)											
Fruit servings	1 (recommended)	2 (recommended for all weight groups)											

Ready reckoner | Weight loss | Females
Up to 12½ stone (79 kg)

	2 restricted days	Less than 8½ stone (54 kg)			8½–9½ stone (54–60 kg)			9½–10½ stone (60–67 kg)			10½–11½ stone (67–73 kg)			11½–12½ stone (73–79 kg)		
		Age 18–29	Age 30–60	Age 60+	Age 18–29	Age 30–60	Age 60+	Age 18–29	Age 30–60	Age 60+	Age 18–29	Age 30–60	Age 60+	Age 18–29	Age 30–60	Age 60+
Maximum kcal per day	1,000	1,500	1,400	1,400	1,500	1,400	1,400	1,700	1,500	1,400	1,800	1,600	1,500	1,900	1,700	1,600
Carbohydrate servings	0	Max 6	Max 6	Max 6	Max 6	Max 6	Max 6	Max 7	Max 6	Max 6	Max 8	Max 7	Max 6	Max 9	Max 7	Max 7
Protein servings	Min 4 / Max 12	Min 3 / Max 8	Min 3 / Max 8	Min 3 / Max 8	Min 4 / Max 8	Min 4 / Max 8	Min 4 / Max 8	Min 5 / Max 10	Min 5 / Max 8	Min 5 / Max 8	Min 6 / Max 11	Min 6 / Max 9	Min 6 / Max 8	Min 7 / Max 12	Min 7 / Max 10	Min 7 / Max 9
Fat servings	Max 5	Max 4	Max 3	Max 3	Max 4	Max 3	Max 3	Max 5	Max 4	Max 3	Max 5	Max 4	Max 4	Max 5	Max 5	Max 4
Dairy servings	3 (recommended)	3 (recommended for all weight groups)														
Vegetable servings	5 (recommended)	5 (recommended for all weight groups)														
Fruit servings	1 (recommended)	2 (recommended for all weight groups)														

Ready reckoner | Weight loss | Females
Over 12½ stone (79 kg)

	2 restricted days	5 unrestricted days											
		12½–13½ stone (79–86 kg)			13½–14½ stone (86–92 kg)			14½–15½ stone (92–98 kg)			Above 15½ stone (98 kg)		
		Age 18–29	Age 30–60	Age 60+	Age 18–29	Age 30–60	Age 60+	Age 18–29	Age 30–60	Age 60+	Age 18–29	Age 30–60	Age 60+
Maximum kcal per day	1,000	2,000	1,800	1,700	2,000	1,900	1,800	2,000	2,000	1,800	2,000	2,000	1,900
Carbohydrate servings	0	Max 9	Max 8	Max 7	Max 9	Max 9	Max 8	Max 9	Max 9	Max 8	Max 9	Max 9	Max 9
Protein servings	Min 4	Min 8	Min 8	Min 8	Min 9	Min 9	Min 9	Min 10	Min 10	Min 10	Min 11	Min 11	Min 11
	Max 12	Max 14	Max 11	Max 10	Max 14	Max 12	Max 11	Max 14	Max 14	Max 11	Max 14	Max 14	Max 12
Fat servings	Max 5	Max 5	Max 5	Max 5	Max 5	Max 5	Max 5	Max 5	Max 5	Max 5	Max 5	Max 5	Max 5
Dairy servings	3 (recommended)	3 (recommended for all weight groups)											
Vegetable servings	5 (recommended)	5 (recommended for all weight groups)											
Fruit servings	1 (recommended)	2 (recommended for all weight groups)											

Ready reckoner | Weight maintenance | Males
Up to 11½ stone (73 kg)

	1 restricted days	Less than 8½ stone (54 kg) Age 18–29	Age 30–60	Age 60+	8½–9½ stone (54–60 kg) Age 18–29	Age 30–60	Age 60+	9½–10½ stone (60–67 kg) Age 18–29	Age 30–60	Age 60+	10½–11½ stone (67–73 kg) Age 18–29	Age 30–60	Age 60+
					6 unrestricted days								
Maximum kcal per day	1,100	1,900	1,800	1,600	2,000	1,900	1,700	2,100	2,000	1,800	2,300	2,200	2,000
Carbohydrate servings	0	Max 8	Max 8	Max 7	Max 9	Max 9	Max 7	Max 11	Max 9	Max 8	Max 12	Max 11	Max 9
Protein servings	Min 4	Min 3	Min 3	Min 3	Min 4	Min 4	Min 4	Min 5	Min 5	Min 5	Min 6	Min 6	Min 6
	Max 14	Max 12	Max 11	Max 9	Max 14	Max 12	Max 10	Max 14	Max 14	Max 11	Max 16	Max 15	Max 14
Fat servings	Max 6	Max 5	Max 5	Max 4	Max 5	Max 5	Max 5	Max 5	Max 5	Max 5	Max 6	Max 5	Max 5
Dairy servings	3 (recommended)	3 (recommended for all weight groups)											
Vegetable servings	5 (recommended)	5 (recommended for all weight groups)											
Fruit servings	1 (recommended)	2 (recommended for all weight groups)											

Ready reckoner | Weight maintenance | Males

Over 11½ stone (73 kg)

	1 restricted days	6 unrestricted days											
		11½–12½ stone (73–79 kg)			12½–13½ stone (79–86 kg)			13½–14½ stone (86–92 kg)			Above 14½ stone (92 kg)		
		Age 18–29	Age 30–60	Age 60+	Age 18–29	Age 30–60	Age 60+	Age 18–29	Age 30–60	Age 60+	Age 18–29	Age 30–60	Age 60+
Maximum kcal per day	1,100	2,400	2,300	2,100	2,500	2,400	2,200	2,500	2,500	2,300	2,500	2,500	2,500
Carbohydrate servings	0	Max 12	Max 12	Max 11	Max 13	Max 12	Max 11	Max 13	Max 13	Max 12	Max 13	Max 13	Max 13
Protein servings	Min 4	Min 7	Min 7	Min 7	Min 8	Min 8	Min 8	Min 9	Min 9	Min 9	Min 10	Min 10	Min 10
	Max 14	Max 17	Max 16	Max 14	Max 17	Max 17	Max 15	Max 17	Max 17	Max 16	Max 17	Max 17	Max 17
Fat servings	Max 6	Max 6	Max 6	Max 5	Max 7	Max 6	Max 5	Max 7	Max 7	Max 6	Max 7	Max 7	Max 7
Dairy servings	3 (recommended)	3 (recommended for all weight groups)											
Vegetable servings	5 (recommended)	5 (recommended for all weight groups)											
Fruit servings	1 (recommended)	2 (recommended for all weight groups)											

Ready reckoner | Weight maintenance | Females
Up to 11½ stone (73 kg)

	1 restricted days	6 unrestricted days											
		Less than 8½ stone (54 kg)			8½–9½ stone (54–60 kg)			9½–10½ stone (60–67 kg)			10½–11½ stone (67–73 kg)		
		Age 18–29	Age 30–60	Age 60+	Age 18–29	Age 30–60	Age 60+	Age 18–29	Age 30–60	Age 60+	Age 18–29	Age 30–60	Age 60+
Maximum kcal per day	1,000	1,700	1,600	1,500	1,800	1,700	1,500	1,900	1,800	1,600	2,000	1,900	1,700
Carbohydrate servings	0	Max 7	Max 7	Max 6	Max 8	Max 7	Max 6	Max 9	Max 8	Max 7	Max 9	Max 9	Max 7
Protein servings	Min 4	Min 3	Min 3	Min 3	Min 4	Min 4	Min 4	Min 5	Min 5	Min 5	Min 6	Min 6	Min 6
	Max 12	Max 10	Max 9	Max 8	Max 11	Max 10	Max 8	Max 12	Max 11	Max 9	Max 14	Max 12	Max 10
Fat servings	Max 5	Max 5	Max 4	Max 4	Max 5	Max 5	Max 4	Max 5	Max 5	Max 4	Max 5	Max 5	Max 5
Dairy servings	3 (recommended)	3 (recommended for all weight groups)											
Vegetable servings	5 (recommended)	5 (recommended for all weight groups)											
Fruit servings	1 (recommended)	2 (recommended for all weight groups)											

Ready reckoner | Weight maintenance | Females

Over 11½ stone (73 kg)

	1 restricted days	6 unrestricted days											
		11½–12½ stone (73–79 kg)			12½–13½ stone (79–86 kg)			13½–14½ stone (86–92 kg)			Above 14½ stone (92 kg)		
		Age 18–29	Age 30–60	Age 60+	Age 18–29	Age 30–60	Age 60+	Age 18–29	Age 30–60	Age 60+	Age 18–29	Age 30–60	Age 60+
Maximum kcal per day	1,000	2,000	1,900	1,800	2,000	2,000	1,900	2,000	2,000	2,000	2,000	2,000	2,000
Carbohydrate servings	0	Max 9	Max 9	Max 8	Max 9	Max 9	Max 9	Max 9	Max 9	Max 9	Max 9	Max 9	Max 9
Protein servings	Min 4	Min 7	Min 7	Min 7	Min 8	Min 8	Min 8	Min 9	Min 9	Min 9	Min 10	Min 10	Min 10
	Max 12	Max 14	Max 12	Max 11	Max 14	Max 14	Max 12	Max 14	Max 14	Max 14	Max 14	Max 14	Max 14
Fat servings	Max 5	Max 5	Max 5	Max 5	Max 5	Max 5	Max 5	Max 5	Max 5	Max 5	Max 5	Max 5	Max 5
Dairy servings	3 (recommended)	3 (recommended for all weight groups)											
Vegetable servings	5 (recommended)	5 (recommended for all weight groups)											
Fruit servings	1 (recommended)	2 (recommended for all weight groups)											

Appendix E: Top 10 fibre-rich foods

The two tables below show the top ten fibre-rich foods for your restricted and unrestricted days[5, 6]. Aim to include as many as possible within your servings allowance.

Food	Serving size		Total fibre (g)	Soluble fibre (g)	insoluble fibre (g)
	description	g			
Restricted days					
Raspberries	1 handful	80	5.5	1.5	4.0
Frozen soya beans	4 tbsp	60	3.7	1.8	1.9
Green beans	4 tbsp	80	2.5	0.6	1.9
Broccoli	2 spears	80	2.4	1.2	1.2
Apricots, dried	3	25	2.2	1.2	1.0
Cauliflower	8 florets	80	2.2	0.9	1.3
Spinach (cooked)	2 tbsp	80	2.2	0.7	1.5
Brussels sprouts	8	80	2.1	1.1	1.0
Flaxseeds	2 tsp	7	1.9	0.6	1.3
Almonds	4 nuts	8	0.8	0.1	0.7
Unrestricted days					
High fibre bran cereal	3 tbsp	24	5.9	1.0	4.9
Raspberries	1 handful	80	5.5	1.5	4.0
Peas	3 tbsp	80	5.4	1.6	3.8
Kidney beans	1 tbsp	40	3.2	0.8	2.4
Bran flakes	3 tbsp	24	3.1	0.3	2.9
Rye crispbread	2	20	3.1	1.3	1.8
Pearl barley	Level tbsp uncooked	20	3.1	0.8	2.3
Figs, ready to eat	3	25	3.0	1.4	1.6
Grape-nuts	3 tbsp	24	2.8	0.8	2.0
Pasta, whole wheat, cooked	2 tbsp	60	2.8	0.6	2.2

Appendix F: How to include more daily physical activity

The chart below shows how you can burn off more calories during the day by simply making some small adjustments to your normal routine. You should aim to combine planned exercise with small amounts of activity during the day for the best results.

Gym day with minimal daily activities	Calories used *	Non gym day with daily activities	Calories used*
Take the bus to work (20 min)	30	Get off the bus 5 min early and walk 15 min	84
Take the lift up 2 floors, 5 times during the day	3	Walk up and down 2 floors, 5 times during the day	54
Email a colleague	8	Walk 2 min to colleague, stand and talk 5 min, walk 2 min back to desk	33
Buy sandwich from trolley	3	Walk to sandwich shop, 5 min each way	35
Take the bus home (20 min)	30	Get off the bus 5 min early and walk 15 min	84
Drive to gym (7 min)	20	Watch television (1 hour)	90
Aerobics class (45 min)	262		
Drive home (7 min)	20		
Reheat ready meal (5 min)	5	Prepare a meal (30 min)	70
Watch television (1 hour 25 min)	128	Vacuum (30 min), iron (30 min)	178
Do online food shopping (30 min)	45	Walk to the shops (15 min each way) Food shopping (30 min)	193
Let the dog out in the garden	2	Walk the dog (30 min)	105
Reading (1 hour 15 min)	115	Reading (15 min)	23
Total calories	671	Total calories	859

*Estimated for an 11 stone (70 kg) woman

Appendix G:
My 12-Week exercise plan

This 12-week walking programme is designed so that you can build up the level of exercise over several weeks. If the first week feels too easy, start at Week 3 or 4; if you're finding it tough, repeat that week until you're ready to move on. Work through the full 12 weeks.

By Week 12 you will be doing 150 minutes moderate exercise, which is about half an hour for five days a week – irrespective of wherever you were at the start. Moderate exercise walking pace is defined as between 4–6.4 kilometres per hour (2½–4 mph) on flat level ground.

Week		1	2	3	4	5	6	7	8	9	10	11	12
Beginner Not currently exercising at all	Time (Min)	5	5	5	10	10	15	15	20	20	25	25	30
	Speed (mph)	1.5	1.5	1.5	1.5	2	2	2	2	2	2	2.5	2.5
	Frequency (Sessions/week)	1	2	3	3	3	4	4	4	5	5	5	5
Intermediate Currently doing at least one exercise session a week	Time (Min)	10	10	10	15	15	20	20	25	25	30	30	30
	Speed (mph)	2	2	2.5	2.5	2.5	2.5	2.5	3	3	3	3	3
	Frequency (Sessions/week)	2	3	3	4	4	4	5	5	5	5	5	5
Advanced Currently doing at least two exercise sessions a week	Time (Min)	15	15	15	20	20	20	25	25	30	30	30	30
	Speed (mph)	3	3	3	3	3	3.5	3.5	3.5	3.5	3.5	4	4
	Frequency (Sessions/week)	3	4	4	5	5	5	5	5	5	5	5	5

It is recommended that you continue to exercise for 150 minutes per week at a moderate level for another 12 weeks and really get the exercise habit stuck before you begin to build to 300 minutes moderate exercise per week.

Once you have completed the 0–150-minute 12-week walking plan you are ready to follow the next 150–300-minute 12-week plan, which you will find at www.thetwodaydiet.co.uk.

FurtherInformation

The 2-Day Diet website
www.thetwodaydiet.co.uk

Healthy lifestyle information
NHS Change for Life (campaign to improve family health):
   www.nhs.uk/Change4Life/Pages/change-for-life.aspx
NHS Live Well (includes couch to 5K information):
   www.nhs.uk/livewell/Pages/Livewellhub.aspx

Health conditions information
Genesis Breast Cancer Prevention research:
   www.genesisuk.org
British Heart Foundation:
   www.bhf.org.uk/heart-health/prevention.aspx
Diabetes UK: www.diabetes.org.uk
Arthritis Care: www.arthritiscare.org.uk

Journal resources
PubMed electronic journal resource:
   www.ncbi.nlm.nih.gov/entrez
Centre for disease control and prevention:
   www.cdc.gov/Publications
NICE (National Institute of Clinical Excellence):
   www.nice.org.uk
UK health statistics:
   www.ons.gov.uk/ons/publications/index.html

Food
Food Standards Agency: www.food.gov.uk
The Nutrition Society: www.nutritionsociety.org/index.asp

Weight Management

British Dietetic Association Weight Wise:
www.bdaweightwise.com

Weight Concern: www.weightconcern.org.uk

National Obesity Forum: www.nationalobesityforum.org.uk

National Heart, Lung and Blood Institute guidelines on
weight management Identification, Evaluation, Treatment
of Overweight and Obesity in Adults: www.nhlbi.nih.gov/
guidelines/obesity/ob_home.htm

Physical Activity

Walking for health: www.walkingforhealth.org.uk

Sports Council for England: www.sportengland.org

Couch to 5K free training app:
www.nhs.uk/LiveWell/c25k/Pages/couch-to-5k.aspx

American College of Sports Medicine: www.acsm.org

Sustrans: www.sustrans.org.uk

Ramblers Association: www.ramblers.org.uk

Fitness and exercise website (commercial): www.netfit.co.uk

Australian Physio Website (commercial):
www.physioadvisor.com

For activities or organisations local to you, try searching via a
search engine or try your local council's website.

references

1. Why The 2-Day Diet works

1. Harvie M, Howell A et al., 'Association of gain and loss of weight before and after menopause with risk of postmenopausal breast cancer in the Iowa women's health study', *Cancer Epidemiology, Biomarkers & Prevention*, 14/3 (2005), 656–61.

2. Wing RR et al., 'Long-term weight loss maintenance', *The American Journal of Clinical Nutrition*, 82/1 Suppl (2005), 222S–225S.

3. http://www.ic.nhs.uk/statistics-and-data-collections/health-and-life-styles-related-surveys/health-survey-for-england/health-survey-for-england--2010-trend-tables

4. http://epp.eurostat.ec.europa.eu/statisticsexplained/index.php/Overweight_and_obesity_-_BMI_statistics

5. Cleary MP et al., 'Weight-cycling decreases incidence and increases latency of mammary tumors to a greater extent than does chronic caloric restriction in mouse mammary tumor virus-transforming growth factor-alpha female mice', *Cancer Epidemiology, Biomarkers & Prevention*, 11/9, (2002), 836–43.

6. Anson RM, Mattson MP et al., 'Intermittent fasting dissociates beneficial effects of dietary restriction on glucose metabolism and neuronal resistance to injury from calorie intake', *Proceedings of the National Academy of Sciences of the United States of America*, 100/10 (2003), 6216–20.

7. Harvie MN, Howell A et al., 'The effects of intermittent or continuous energy restriction on weight loss and metabolic disease risk markers: a randomized trial in young overweight women', *International Journal of Obesity* (London), 35/5 (2011), 714–27.

8. Harvie MN, Howell A et al., P3–09–02: 'Intermittent Dietary Carbohydrate Restriction Enables Weight Loss and Reduces Breast Cancer Risk Biomarkers', Thirty-Fourth Annual CTRC-AACR San Antonio Breast Cancer Symposium (San Antonio, TX) (6–10 Dec, 2011).

9. Veldhorst MA et al., 'Presence or absence of carbohydrates and the proportion of fat in a high-protein diet affect appetite suppression but not energy expenditure in normal-weight human subjects fed in energy balance', *British Journal of Nutrition*, 104/9 (2010), 1395–1405.

10. Johnson F et al., 'Dietary restraint and self-regulation in eating behavior', *International Journal of Obesity* (London), 36/5 (2012), 665–674.

11. Jacobsen SC et al., 'Effects of short-term high-fat overfeeding on genome-wide DNA methylation in the skeletal muscle of healthy young men', *Diabetologia*, 12 (2012), 3341–9.

12. Timmers S et al., Calorie restriction-like effects of 30 days of resveratrol supplementation on energy metabolism and metabolic profile in obese humans', *Cell Metabolism*, 14/5 (2011), 612–22.

13. Peeters A et al., 'Obesity in adulthood and its consequences for life expectancy: a life-table analysis', *Annals of Internal Medicine*, 138/1 (2003), 24–32.

14. http://www.ons.gov.uk/ons/rel/disability-and-health-measurement/health-expectancies-at-birth-and-age-65-in-the-united-kingdom/2008–10/index.html

15. Carlson O et al., 'Impact of reduced meal frequency without caloric restriction on glucose regulation in healthy, normal-weight middle-aged men and women', *Metabolism*, 56/12 (2007), 1729–1734.

16. Sandholt CH et al., 'Beyond the fourth wave of genome-wide obesity association studies', *Nutrition & Diabetes*, 2/e37 (2012).

17. Garaulet M et al., 'CLOCK gene is implicated in weight reduction in obese patients participating in a dietary programme based on the Mediterranean diet', *International Journal of Obesity* (London), 34/3 (2010), 516–523.

18. Matsuo T et al., 'Effects of FTO genotype on weight loss and metabolic risk factors in response to calorie restriction among Japanese women', *Obesity* (Silver Spring), 20/5 (2012), 1122–1126.

19. Lovelady C., 'Balancing exercise and food intake with lactation to promote post-partum weight loss', Proceedings of the Nutrition Society, 70/2 (2011), 181–184.

20. http://bda.uk.com/news/news.php

2. Do I Need to Lose Weight?

1. Shea JL et al., 'Body fat percentage is associated with cardiometabolic dysregulation in BMI-defined normal weight subjects', *Nutrition, Metabolism & Cardiovascular Diseases*, 22/9 (2012), 741–747.

2. Sternfeld B et al., 'Changes over 14 years in androgenicity and body mass index in a biracial cohort of reproductive-age women', *The Journal of Clinical Endocrinology & Metabolism*, 93/6 (2008), 2158–65.

3. Harvie MN, Howell AH et al., 'Central obesity and breast cancer risk: a systematic review', *Obesity Reviews*, 4/3 (2003), 157–73.

4. Beck RJ. et al., 'Choral singing, performance perception, and immune system changes in salivary immunoglobulin A and cortisol', *Music Perception*, 18 (1999), 87–106.

5. Nackers LM et al., 'The association between rate of initial weight loss and long-term success in obesity treatment: does slow and steady win the race?' *International Journal of Behavioral Medicine*, 17/3 (2010), 161–167.

6. Paulweber B et al., 'A European evidence-based guideline for the prevention of type 2 diabetes', *Hormone and Metabolic Research*, 42 Suppl 1 (2010), S3–36.

7. Maruthur NM et al., 'Lifestyle interventions reduce coronary heart disease risk: results from the PREMIER Trial', *Circulation*, 119/15 (2009), 2026–2031.

8. Harvie MN, Howell A et al., 'Association of gain and loss of weight before and after menopause with risk of postmenopausal breast cancer in the Iowa women's health study', *Cancer Epidemiology, Biomarkers & Prevention*, 14/3 (2005), 656–661.

9. Larson-Meyer DE et al., 'Effect of calorie restriction with or without exercise on insulin sensitivity, beta-cell function, fat cell size, and ectopic lipid in overweight subjects', *Diabetes Care*, 29/6 (2006), 1337–44.

3. How to do the 2 restricted days

1. Pearce KL, et al., 'Egg consumption as part of an energy-restricted high-protein diet improves blood lipid and blood glucose profiles in individuals with type 2 diabetes', *British Journal of Nutrition*, 105/4 (2011), 584–92.

2. Lieberman HR et al., 'A double-blind, placebo-controlled test of 2 d of calorie deprivation: effects on cognition, activity, sleep, and interstitial glucose concentrations', *The American Journal of Clinical Nutrition*, 88/3 (2008), 667–676.

3. Brinkworth GD et al., 'Long-term effects of a very low-carbohydrate diet and a low-fat diet on mood and cognitive function', *Archives of Internal Medicine*, 169/20 (2009), 1873–1880.

4. Krikorian R et al., 'Dietary ketosis enhances memory in mild cognitive impairment', *Neurobiology Aging*, 33/2 (2012), 425–427.

4. How to eat on the five unrestricted days

1. Willett WC, 'The Mediterranean Diet: Science and practice', *Public Health Nutr*, 9/1A (2006), 105–10.

2. Sevastianova K et al., 'Effect of short-term carbohydrate overfeeding and long-term weight loss on liver fat in overweight humans', *The American Journal of Clinical Nutrition*, 96/4 (2012), 727–34.

3. Bofetta J et al., 'Fruit and vegetable intake and overall cancer risk in the

European Prospective Investigation into Cancer and Nutrition (EPIC)', *Journal of the National Cancer Institute*, 102/8 (2010), 529–37.

4.   Houchins JA et al., 'Effects of fruit and vegetable, consumed in solid vs. beverage forms, on acute and chronic appetitive responses in lean and obese adults', *International Journal of Obesity* (London) (20 Nov 2012).

5.   Stookey JD et al., 'Drinking water is associated with weight loss in overweight dieting women independent of diet and activity', *Obesity* (Silver Spring), 16/11 (2008), 2481–2488.

6.   Flood-Obbagy JE et al., 'The effect of fruit in different forms on energy intake and satiety at a meal', *Appetite*, 52/2 (2009), 416–422.

7.   Backhed F, 'Host responses to the human microbiome', *Nutrition Reviews*, 70 Suppl 1 (2012), S14–S17.

8.   http://www.dh.gov.uk/health/2012/06/sodium-intakes/

9.   Aune D, 'Soft drinks, aspartame and the risk of cancer and cardio-vascular disease', *The American Journal of Clinical Nutrition*, 96/6 (2012), 1249–51.

10.   Chapman CD, et al., 'Lifestyle determinants of the drive to eat: a meta-analysis', *The American Journal of Clinical Nutrition*, 96/3 (2012), 492–7.

11.   Chobanian AV, et al., 'Seventh report of the Joint National Committee on Prevention, Detection, Evaluation, and Treatment of High Blood Pressure', *Hypertension*, 42/6 (2003), 1206–1252.

12.   Nawrot P et al., 'Effects of caffeine on human health', Food Additives and Contaminants, 20/1 (2003), 1–30.

13.   Almoosawi S, et al., 'The effect of polyphenol-rich dark chocolate on fasting capillary whole blood glucose, total cholesterol, blood pressure and glucocorticoids in healthy overweight and obese subjects', *British Journal of Nutrition*, 103/6 (2010), 842–850.

5. Making The 2-Day Diet work

1.   Wansink B, 'Environmental factors that unknowingly influence the consumption and intake of consumers', *Annual Review of Nutrition*, 24 (2004), 455–479.

2.   Dennis EA, et al., 'Water consumption increases weight loss during a hypocaloric diet intervention in middle-aged and older adults', *Obesity* (Silver Spring), 18/2 (2010), 300–7.

3.   Rolls BJ et al., 'The effect of large portion sizes on energy intake is sustained for 11 days', *Obesity*, 15/6 (2007), 1535–43.

4.   Rolls BJ et al., 'Reductions in portion size and energy density of foods are additive and lead to sustained decreases in energy intake', *The American Journal of Clinical Nutrition*, 83/1 (2006), 11–7.

5. Bellisle F, 'Cognitive restraint can be offset by distraction, leading to increased meal intake in women', *The American Journal of Clinical Nutrition*, 74/2 (2001), 197–200.

6. Hirsch, AR et al., 'Effect of Television Viewing on Sensory-Specific Satiety: Are Leno and Letterman Obesogenic?', 89th Annual Meeting Endocrine Society (Abstract) (2007).

7. Byrne NM et al., 'Does metabolic compensation explain the majority of less-than-expected weight loss in obese adults during a short-term severe diet and exercise intervention?' *International Journal of Obesity*, 36/11 (2012), 1472–1478.

8. Bellisle F et al., 'Meal frequency and energy balance', *British Journal of Nutrition*, 77/1 (1997), S57–70.

9. Holmback U et al., 'The human body may buffer small differences in meal size and timing during a 24-hour wake period provided energy balance is maintained', *Journal of Nutrition*, 133/9 (2003), 2748–55.

10. Nedeltcheva, AV et al., 'Sleep curtailment is accompanied by increased intake of calories from snacks', *The American Journal of Clinical Nutrition*, 89 (2009), 126–133.

11. Buxton OM et al., 'Adverse metabolic consequences in humans of prolonged sleep restriction combined with circadian disruption', Science Translational Medicine, 4/129 (2012), 12.

12. Morgan PJ et al., 'Efficacy of a workplace-based weight loss program for overweight male shift workers: the Workplace POWER (Preventing Obesity Without Eating like a Rabbit) randomized controlled trial. *Preventive Medicine*, 52/5 (2011), 317–25.

13. Halsey LG et al., 'Does consuming breakfast influence activity levels? An experiment into the effect of breakfast consumption on eating habits and energy expenditure', *Public Health Nutrition*, 15/2 (2012), 238–245.

14. Ratliff J et al., 'Consuming eggs for breakfast influences plasma glucose and ghrelin, while reducing energy intake during the next 24 hours in adult men', *Nutrition Research*, 30/2 (2010), 96–1003.

15. Mason C et al., 'History of weight cycling does not impede future weight loss or metabolic improvements in postmenopausal women', *Metabolism*, 62/1 (2013), 127–36.

16. Smeets AJ et al., 'Acute effects on metabolism and appetite profile of one meal difference in the lower range of meal frequency', *British Journal of Nutrition*, 99/6 (2008), 1316–1321.

17. Wing RR et al., 'Prescribed "breaks" as a means to disrupt weight control efforts', *Obesity Research*, 11/2 (2003), 287–291.

18. May et al., 'Elaborated Intrusion Theory: A Cognitive-Emotional Theory of Food Craving', *Current Obesity Reports*, 1 (2012), 114–121.

19. Campagne DM, 'The premenstrual syndrome revisited', *European Journal of Obstetrics & Gynecology and Reproductive Biology*, 130/1 (2007), 4–17.

6. How to be more active

1. Redman LM et al., 'Metabolic and behavioral compensations in response to caloric restriction: implications for the maintenance of weight loss', *PLoS One* 4, e4377 (2009).

2. Garrow JS et al., 'Meta-analysis: effect of exercise, with or without dieting, on the body composition of overweight subjects', *European Journal of Clinical Nutrition*, 49 (1995), 1–10.

3. Gill JM et al., 'Exercise and postprandial lipid metabolism: an update on potential mechanisms and interactions with high-carbohydrate diets (review)'. *The Journal of Nutritional Biochemistry*, 14/3 (2003), 122–32.

4. Byberg L et al., 'Total mortality after changes in leisure time physical activity in 50 year old men: 35 year follow-up of population based cohort', *BMJ* 338 (2009), b688.

5. © Canadian Society for Exercise Physiology PAR-Q, www.csep.ca

6. Wilmot EG et al., 'Sedentary time in adults and the association with diabetes, cardiovascular disease and death: systematic review and meta-analysis', *Diabetologia* 55 (2012), 2895–2905.

7. Dunstan DW et al., 'Breaking up prolonged sitting reduces postprandial glucose and insulin responses', *Diabetes Care*, 35/5 (2012), 976–83.

8. O'Donovan et al., 'The ABC of Physical Activity for Health: a consensus statement from the British Association of Sport and Exercise Sciences', *Journal of Sports Sciences*, 28/6 (2010), 573–91.

9. King NA et al., 'Individual variability following 12 weeks of supervised exercise: identification and characterization of compensation for exercise-induced weight loss'. *International Journal of Obesity*, 32 (2008), 177–184.

10. Ainsworth BE et al., '2011 Compendium of Physical Activities: a second update of codes and MET values', *Medicine and Science in Sports and Exercise*, 43/8 (2011), 1575–1581.

11. Ismail I et al., 'A systematic review and meta-analysis of the effect of aerobic vs. resistance exercise training on visceral fat', *Obesity Reviews*, 13/1 (2012), 68–91.

12. Brinkworth GD et al., 'Effects of a low carbohydrate weight loss diet on exercise capacity and tolerance in obese subjects'. *Obesity* (Silver Spring), 17/10 (2009), 1916–1923.

13. Farah NM et al., 'Effects of exercise before or after meal ingestion on fat balance and postprandial metabolism in overweight men', *British Journal of Nutrition* (26 Oct 2012) 1–11.

7. How to stay slim

1.   Sumithran Pet al., 'Long-term persistence of hormonal adaptations to weight loss', *The New England Journal of Medicine*, 365/17 (2011), 1597–1604.

2.   Baldwin KM et al., 'Effects of weight loss and leptin on skeletal muscle in human subjects', *The American Journal of Physiology – Regulatory, Integrative and Comparative Physiology*, 301/5 (2011), R1259–R1266.

3.   Hall KD et al., 'Quantification of the effect of energy imbalance on bodyweight', *The Lancet*, 378/9793 (2011), 826–837.

Appendices

1.   Gomez-Ambrosi J, Silva C, Catalan V, Rodriguez A, Galofre JC, Escalada J et al., 'Clinical usefulness of a new equation for estimating body fat', *Diabetes Care*, 35/2 (2012), 383–388.

2.   Shea JL, King MT, Yi Y, Gulliver W, Sun G., 'Body fat percentage is associated with cardiometabolic dysregulation in BMI-defined normal weight subjects', *Nutrition, Metabolism & Cardiovascular Diseases*, 229 (2012), 741–747.

3.   Henry Basal, CJK, 'Metabolic rate studies in humans: measurement and development of new equations', *Public Health Nutrition*, 8/7a (2005), 1133–1152.

4.   Krieger JW et al., 'Effects of variation in protein and carbohydrate intake on body mass and composition during energy restriction: a meta-regression' *The American Journal of Clinical Nutrition* 83/2 (2006), 260–274.

5.   http://huhs.harvard.edu/assets/file/ourservices/service_nutrition_fiber.pdf

6.   *Plant Fiber in Foods* (2nd ed., 1990) (HCF Nutrition Research Foundation Inc., PO Box 22124, Lexington, KY 40522).

acknowledgements

Many thanks to Anne Montague, Jo Godfrey Wood and Mary Pegington for editing the manuscript; Kate Santon and Emily Jonzen for devising the recipes; Paula Stavrinos for her recipe ideas and Kath Sellers for analysing and collating the recipes for the book. Thanks also to Debbie McMullan and Rebecca Dodd-Chandler for their advice and expertise for the exercise chapter and the illustrator, Stephen Dew.

This book has evolved from our research to date on intermittent diets for weight loss and reducing the risk of disease. We therefore thank our collaborators and colleagues who have made this work possible. Firstly Mark Mattson from the National Institute on Ageing, Baltimore, and Margot Cleary from The University of Minnesota for sharing the insights from their research, which inspired us to undertake our dietary studies. Secondly the team of scientists and researchers who have helped us run these studies: Gareth Evans, Claire Wright, Ellen Mitchell, Helen Sumner, Rosemary Greenhalgh, Jenny Affen, Jayne Beesley at The Nightingale Centre and Genesis Breast Cancer Prevention. We are grateful to the rest of Mark Mattson's team including Bronwen Martin and Roy Cutler, Jan Frystyk and Alan Flyvbjerg (Arhus University Hospital, Denmark), Roy Goodacre, Andrew Vaughan, Will Allwood, Robert Clarke, Kath Spence (all University of Manchester), Andy Sims (University of Edinburgh), Wendy Russell (Rowett Institute) who have all helped to assess the impact of the diets on the body and disease risk. Thanks also to the following individuals for their invaluable advice: Susan Jebb (weight management), Julie Morris (statistics) and Louise Donnelly (health psychology and dieting behaviours).

Our greatest thanks are to Lester Barr, Pam Glass and the Genesis Breast Cancer Prevention trustees who have consistently supported our dietary research for the past 11 years. Also Nikki Hoffman, Michelle Cohen, the Genesis office team and the Genesis volunteers who give up their time to help us in the office and run research clinics, particularly Jane Eaton, Susan Roe, Pauline Sadler, Philippa Quirk, Louise Blacklock, Alison Rees and Angela Foster. Thanks also to Amy Tao and Matthew Collier, our Genesis graduate interns.

We thank the numerous dieters who have worked with us on the studies over the past 11 years, without whom none of the research would be possible, and staff within The Nightingale Centre and Genesis Breast Cancer Prevention who have been successfully dieting with our 2-Day Diet and inspired us to write this book.

Finally Susanna Abbott and Catherine Knight at Ebury for their patience and hard work in making this book.

index